Atlas of the
Peripheral Ocular Fundus

Atlas of the
Peripheral Ocular Fundus

William L. Jones
Chief of Optometry
Veterans Administration Medical Center
Albuquerque, New Mexico

Clinical Instructor
School of Medicine
University of New Mexico

Robert W. Reidy
Chief of Ophthalmology
Chief of Retinal Services
School of Medicine
University of New Mexico

Butterworth Publishers

Boston • London
Sydney • Wellington • Durban • Toronto

To our wives, Siu and Kathy, and our families for all their support during the writing of this book

Library of Congress Cataloging in Publication Data

Jones, William L., 1946–
    Atlas of the peripheral ocular fundus.

    Includes index.
    1. Fundus oculi—Diseases—Atlases. I. Reidy, Robert W. II. Title.
RE545.J66 1984   617.7′4   84–14984
ISBN 0–409–95174–9

Butterworth Publishers
80 Montvale Avenue
Stoneham, MA 02180

10 9 8 7 6 5 4 3

Printed in the United States of America

Contents

Preface

This book was designed to be a readily available source on the peripheral ocular fundus for eye care practitioners. It covers many of the developmental anomalies of the peripheral retina, ora serrata, and pars plana, but emphasis is placed on anomalies and degenerations of the retina and vitreous, which have the potential for producing a retinal break or detachment. A detailed discussion of each entity includes clinical description, histopathology, clinical significance, and brief suggestions for treatment.

Each condition is represented by photographs, most of which were taken through the condensing lens used for binocular indirect ophthalmoscopy. This technique produces a picture free of many of the distortions seen in photographs taken with a standard fundus camera. The realistic view of the peripheral ocular fundus will allow clinicians to greatly enhance their perception and understanding of peripheral fundus lesions. There are many diagrammatic representations that simplify the pathologic characteristics of each lesion and significantly enhance the readers' comprehension of their clinical and pathologic appearance. There are also a number of B-scan ultrasonograms to enhance the description of these entities.

W.L. Jones
R.W. Reidy

1 Viewing the Peripheral Fundus

Figure 1.1 Pocket clip and thimble scleral depressors.

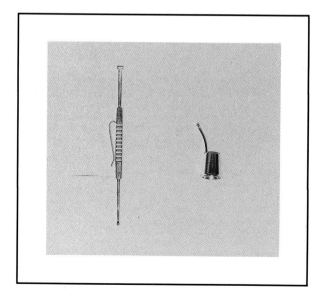

To view the peripheral fundus adequately requires that the pupil be dilated and necessitates the use of an indirect ophthalmoscope. Good dilation is usually achieved by instilling one drop of tropicamide (Mydriacyl) 1% and phenylephrine (Neosynephrine) 2.5% and waiting 20 to 30 minutes for the drugs to take effect. An adequate view of the intraocular structures anterior to the equator requires the use of an indirect ophthalmoscope, either a monocular or a binocular indirect ophthalmoscope. The monocular indirect ophthalmoscope has the advantages of being easy to use and providing good magnification and an erect image. The disadvantages are that the viewer cannot see as far peripherally as with a binocular indirect scope, it is very difficult to perform scleral depression, and there is no stereopsis to help detect depressed or elevated lesions.

Binocular indirect ophthalmoscopes deliver a large field of view at the expense of magnification; however, most lesions of the peripheral fundus can be easily seen with this method. Its other advantages are stereopsis, a bright light source, and the ability to see very peripheral lesions with the aid of scleral depression. The disadvantages of the binocular indirect ophthalmoscope are that it demands a greater degree of skill to use and the image produced by the condensing lens is reversed and inverted. The binocular indirect ophthalmoscope is the instrument of choice for examining the peripheral fundus.

Scleral depressors are used to indent the globe. They are constructed of stainless steel-plated metal in either a straight or curved configuration; some even have a thimble cup arrangement (Figure 1.1). Scleral depression can be accomplished by depressing either through the lids or upon the bulbar conjunctiva after administering topical anesthesia. It is usually not necessary to apply inward pressure; all that is generally needed to achieve adequate depression is to insert the depressor into the orbit adjacent to the globe. Scleral depression through the lids usually produces little discomfort, and topical anesthesia is not required. If a metal depressor is not available, a cotton-tipped applicator is a good substitute. When performing this procedure, care should be taken not to cause a corneal abrasion by rubbing the cornea with the depressor. The metal depressor should be cleaned with soapy water or alcohol after each use.

Scleral depression pushes peripheral fundus structures into the viewing and illumination beams of the ophthalmoscope (Figure 1.2).

Figure 1.2 Scleral depression. Note that depressing the globe, through the eyelid in this case, pushes the peripheral retina into view. Courtesy of Matthew Garston and Anthony Cavallerano, Review of Optometry 1979; 116:81—84.

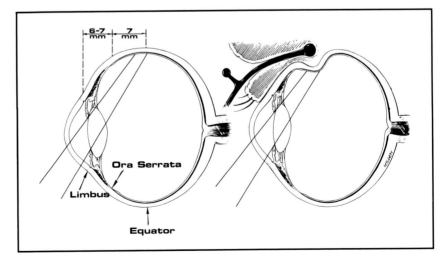

With this technique, it is possible to see from the ora serrata to the tips of the ciliary processes. During the actual indenting of the globe, a "roll" of retina or pars plana is produced. Moving the depressor back and forth causes a lesion to be moved higher or lower on the roll so that it can be viewed at different angles of illumination and on edge. This is helpful in the diagnosis of a retinal break as it allows the clinician a view of its edge (see Figures 3.49 and 3.54, pages 69 and 86). As far as we are aware, scleral depression has not initiated or exacerbated a retinal detachment when it is performed to evaluate a peripheral fundus lesion.

The Goldmann three-mirror contact lens can also be used with the biomicroscope to view the peripheral fundus. Its advantages are magnification, stereopsis, and the lack of mirror image reversing. Disadvantages are contact with the globe, which requires significant patient cooperation, and a smaller field of view.

2 Anatomy of the Peripheral Fundus

Retina

The retina is composed of the inner neural or sensory layers and the outer pigment epithelium (refer to Figure 2.1 for this discussion). There are nine layers of the neural retina; from inner to outer they are the internal limiting membrane, nerve fiber layer, ganglion cell layer, inner plexiform layer, inner nuclear layer, outer plexiform layer, outer nuclear layer, external limiting membrane, and photoreceptors. The normal neural retina is essentially transparent except for the pigment in the blood, although it does absorb a small quantity of light passing through it. The pigment epithelium generally varies from light gray to jet black (as seen in pigment epithelial hypertrophy or hyperplasia) (see Chapter 3, page 26). Melanin is responsible for its blackish color, and it also contains lipofuscin, a wear-and-tear pigment that has a golden orange color. In minuscule quantities, as in a blonde fundus, the pigment epithelium appears to be essentially transparent (Figure 2.2).

Figure 2.1   Diagrammatic representation of normal
retina.

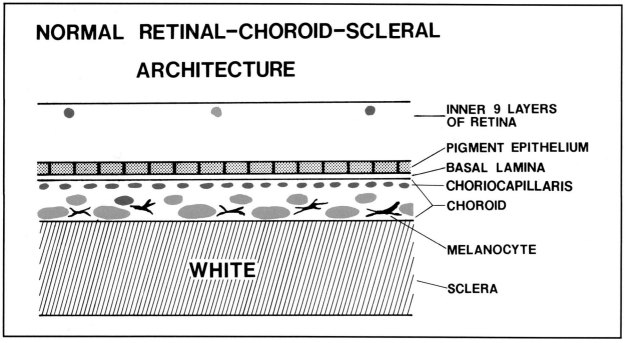

Choroid

The choroid is made up of many layers; the innermost is the basal lamina (Bruch's membrane), which is thin and essentially transparent. The layer below the basal lamina is the choriocapillaris, composed of a fine meshwork of interlacing large capillaries that result in a bright red color. The layer of medium and large choroidal vessels is immediately below the choriocapillaris. The vessels add to the reddish color of the choroid; however, they do not form a uniform red filter, as does the choriocapillaris. Among the medium and large vessels can be found melanocytes, which give the choroid a blackish color. Again, melanin is responsible for the black color. Finally, there is the sclera, which is white.

The bright orange to grayish color of the fundus reflex depends on hemoglobin in the blood vessels and on the amount of melanin in the pigment epithelium and the choroidal melanocytes. The appearance of many lesions of the peripheral fundus depends on which of the pigmented structures is exaggerated or missing. A studious examination and understanding of Figure 2.1 will greatly enhance the clinician's understanding of diseases affecting the peripheral fundus.

Equator

The equator of the fundus is approximately 14 to 15 mm from the limbus and can be located by finding the vortex veins (Figures 2.2 and 2.3). The vortex system is composed of tributaries that vary in size and shape and generally number between 4 and 15.[1] They empty into the ampulla, the dilated sac of the vortex vein, which may have a pigmented crescent. The vortex veins travel obliquely through scleral canals for approximately 4 mm and exit the globe posterior to the equator. There are usually four vortex veins (one per quadrant): the superior veins drain into the superior ophthalmic vein and the inferior veins into the inferior ophthalmic vein. There have been instances where as many as eight to ten vortex veins were found in one eye. The equator can be visualized by drawing an imaginary circle through the ampullae of the vortex veins.

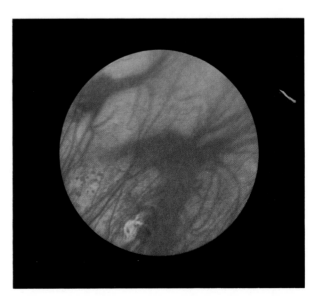

Figure 2.2 Vortex vein seen in a blond fundus. Note the tributaries, the ampula, and the exiting vein that disappears into the sclera. Small pigmented areas are the result of hyperplasia of the pigment epithelium.

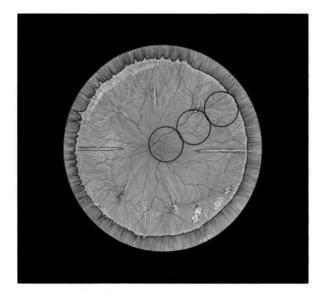

Figure 2.3   The peripheral fundus. The three black circles represent the views through an 18-diopter condensing lens from the optic disc to the ora serrata. The long ciliary nerves and long posterior ciliary arteries are seen at the 3 and 9 o'clock positions. Short ciliary nerves are seen at 1:30, 2, 6:30, and 11:30 o'clock. A large ora tooth is at 10 o'clock and double ora teeth are seen at 11 o'clock. There are five vortex veins located at 2, 5:30, 7:30, 10, and 11:30, and some show pigmentation at the site of the ampula. Peripheral cystoid degeneration is seen circumferentially next to the ora serrata. Chorioretinal atrophy is seen from 4 to 5 o'clock and white-without-pressure is seen from 9:30 to 12 o'clock. A retinal tuft with vitreous traction is seen at 8 o'clock. There is pigment cuffing of a retinal venule at 4 o'clock. The pars plana is the light brown broad ring peripheral to the ora serrata. Courtesy of Matthew Garston and Anthony Cavallerano, Review of Optometry 1979;116:43–49.

Ciliary Nerves and Arteries

Long and short ciliary nerves run perpendicular to the ora serrata in the peripheral fundus (Figure 2.4). They are initially seen approximately at the equator and usually disappear from view at the ora serrata. They are located in the suprachoroidal space. Two long ciliary nerves are found at the medial and temporal aspects of the globe (Figure 2.3) and thus divided the fundus into superior and inferior halves. The short ciliary nerves number from 10 to 20 and are found at locations in the fundus other than the 3 and 9 o'clock positions (Figure 2.3). Both the long and short ciliary nerves may have pigmented margins.

The nasal long posterior ciliary artery is located just superior to the nasal long ciliary nerve, and the temporal long posterior ciliary artery is just inferior to the temporal long ciliary nerve (Figure 2.3). The short posterior ciliary arteries are seen at other locations in the fundus. As with the ciliary nerves, the arteries may also have pigmented margins.

Retinal blood vessels become smaller and more numerous as they travel from the posterior pole into the peripheral retina. Arterioles are

Figure 2.4 The nasal long ciliary nerve seen through the indirect condensing lens.

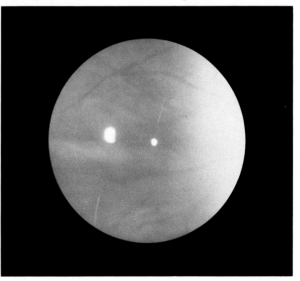

smaller in caliber and lighter in color than the venules. Retinal vessels may even travel parallel to the ora serrata in the far periphery. Most of the blood vessels seem to disappear approximately 2 mm from the ora serrata.

Anterior to the equator is the peripheral retina, which is approximately three disc diameters in width and ends at the ora serrata. Almost all peripheral retinal lesions discussed in this text are located in this zone.

Ora Serrata

The ora serrata denotes the anterior limit of the neural retina. As the neural retina approaches the ora, there is loss of the ganglion and nerve fiber layers, merging of the inner and outer nuclear layers, and loss of photoreceptors. The inner limiting membrane interweaves with the vitreous base and the external limiting membrane continues into the ciliary body as a junctional zone betwen the pigmented and the nonpigmented epithelia. The residual sensory retina continues forward as the nonpigmented epithelium. The retinal pigment epithelium continues forward as the pigmented epithelium of the ciliary body.

The ora serrata is a scalloped-appearing structure, serrated more nasally than temporally (Figure 2.3). It is 2 mm wide nasally and 1 mm wide temporally. It is slightly anterior nasally, 7 mm from the nasal limbus as compared to 8 mm from the temporal limbus. This corresponds to the insertion of the medial and lateral rectus muscles. The rounded extensions of the pars

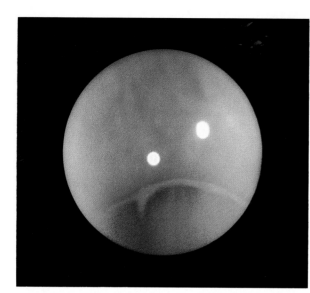

Figure 2.5 The superior ora serrata shows two ora bays and an ora tooth seen through the indirect condensing lens with scleral depression.

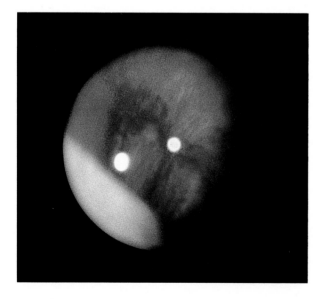

plana at the ora serrata are called ora bays, and the retinal extensions in between the bays are known as dentate processes or ora teeth (Figures 2.3, 2.5, and 2.6). There are approximately 20 to 30 dentate processes per eye. An anatomic variation of the pars plana at the ora serrata is the finding of a deep ora bay (Figure 2.7) or a large ora tooth (Figure 2.3). Deep ora bays are found at least six times more frequently than any other variation of the ora serrata, they have a tendency to be bilateral, and are two to four times wider than adjacent bays.[2] Generally, there is an absence of bays and teeth on the temporal ora serrata. This is due to a difference in the development of the temporal pars plana as compared to the nasal half. Another developmental variation is a bridging ora tooth which is not in contact with the ciliary epithelium of the pars plana and thus forms a curved bridgelike structure. It extends from the peripheral retina to as far anterior as the middle of the pars plana. It often displays a marked degree of cystoid degeneration.[2]

The transition between the more and less scalloped ora serrata is slightly temporal to the 12 o'clock meridian superiorly and slightly nasal to the 6 o'clock meridian inferiorly. A vertical line drawn between these two points is called the anatomical meridian and marks the watershed drainage of the temporal and nasal vortex vein collection systems.[2] The average ora serrata has 16 dentate processes, 1 large or giant dentate process, 10 ora bays, and 1 double ora bay.[3,4] The ora serrata is the anterior limit of a retinal detachment.

Figure 2.6 The superior ora serrata shows three ora bays and prominent retinal pigmentation just posterior to the ora, which denotes the location of the vitreous base. The view is through an indirect condensing lens with scleral depression.

Figure 2.7 The nasal ora serrata shows a deep ora bay and white-with-pressure seen through the indirect condensing lens with scleral depression.

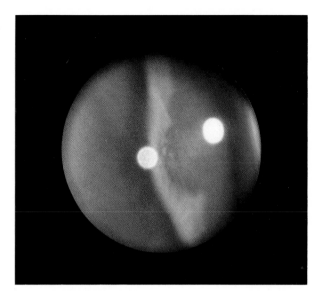

Pars Plana

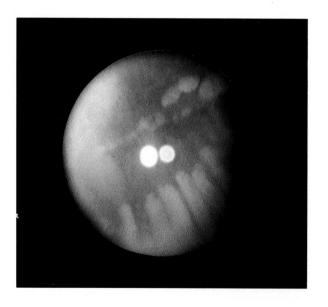

The pars plana is a broad, pigmented, chocolate-colored band that stretches from the pars ciliaris to the ora serrata (Figures 2.3 and 2.8). It is composed of an inner nonpigmented epithelium, an outer pigmented epithelium, basal lamina, and a layer of blood vessels. The pars plana is approximately 4 mm wide nasally and 5 mm wide temporally. There can be a detachment of the nonpigmented epithelium from the pigmented epithelium (see Figure 3.3, page 23).

Figure 2.8   View of the superior peripheral fundus shows from top to bottom: peripheral retina with paving-stone degeneration, ora serrata, pars plana, and the tips of the ciliary processes, which appear as whitish, fingerlike projections. The view is through an indirect condensing lens in an eye with a sector iridectomy.

Corona Ciliaris

The corona ciliaris is the anterior portion of the ciliary body and is approximately 2 mm wide. It contains approximately 60 to 70 ciliary processes that appear a light cream color when seen during indirect ophthalmoscopy (Figure 2.8). The color is created when the nonpigmented epithelium is seen on the internal surface of the processes with tangential illumination. Ciliary processes seen with straight-on illumination through a peripheral iridectomy or iridodialysis during gonioscopy are brown because of the pigment epithelium under the nonpigmented epithelium. The corona ciliaris is composed of nonpigmented and pigmented epithelia, stroma, blood vessels, and smooth muscle.

Vitreous Base

Figure 2.9 Anterior margin of vitreous base can be seen as a white line half way up on the pars plana (arrow). The temporal ora serrata is in view through the indirect condensing lens with scleral depression.

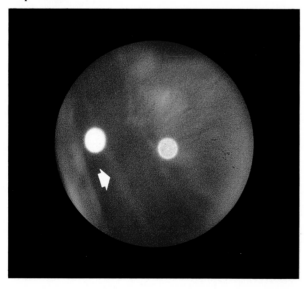

The vitreous base or vitreoretinal symphysis is a 2- to 3-mm band that straddles the ora serrata and is wider nasally than temporally. The anterior limit is sometimes seen as a whitish ridge on the pars plana (Figure 2.9). The posterior margin usually cannot be seen; however, its anterior and posterior limits are often denoted by an increase in pigmentation of ciliary body and retinal pigment epthelium beneath the vitreous base (Figure 2.6). This increased pigmentation is possibly the result of irritation to the pigment epithelium from vitreous traction on the base. The posterior margin of the vitreous base may become visible under severe vitreous traction and appears as a thin, elevated, whitish ridge. The vitreous base is the dividing line between the anterior and posterior vitreous cortex.

A dense network of vitreous fibrils originates in the base. The fibrils penetrate to the basal lamina of the nonpigmented epithelium of the pars plana. The internal limiting membrane of the retina is absent under the symphysis and the vitreous fibrils form intricate bonds with the retinal glial cells. The vitreous base is the most adherent location of the vitreous to the internal surface of the globe, and any attempt to pull it free results in a tearing of the nonpigmented epithelium of the pars plana or retinal tissue. A posterior vitreous detachment usually stops at the posterior margin of the base, which denotes its location.

With age, the posterior margin of the vitreous base may develop posterior extensions as far back as the equator, and it is common to find retinal breaks at these extensions. Approximately 15% of breaks are found along irregularities in the posterior margin of the vitreous base.[5] When a retinal tear occurs just posterior to this margin, the physical ripping stops at the vitreous base and denotes its location (See Figure 5.9, page 160). If the posterior margin of the vitreous base corresponds to the ora serrata and a tear develops there, a retinal dialysis is produced. A large break along the posterior edge of the base is known as a giant retinal tear. Tears can also occur on the pars plana at the anterior margin of the base; they tend to be linear or triangular in shape. These may lead to a detachment of the nonpigmented from the pigmented epithelium.

REFERENCES

1. Cavallerano A, Garston MJ. Examination of the peripheral ocular fundus. Rev Optom 1979; 11:43–49.
2. Rutnin U. Fundus appearance in normal eyes. Parts I and II. Am J Ophthalmol 1967;64:821–852.
3. Straatsma BR, Foos FY, et al. The retina—topography and clinical correlations. In: New Orleans Academy of Ophthalmology: symposium on retina and retinal surgery. St. Louis: CV Mosby, 1969.
4. Straatsma BR, Landers MB, et al. The ora serrata in the adult human eye. Arch Ophthalmol 1968;80:3–20.
5. Schepens CL. Retinal detachment and allied diseases. Philadelphia: WB Saunders, 1983:186.

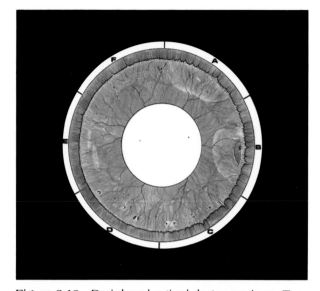

Figure 2.10 Peripheral retinal degenerations. Typical lattice degeneration is seen between 10:30 and 12 o'clock; the lattice at 5 o'clock has a hole within the lesion and a small tear at the nasal edge. Two retinoschisis cavities are seen between 12 and 4 o'clock. The upper retinoschisis has snowflakes along its posterior margin and a thin pigmented demarcation line at its inferior nasal margin. The lower retinoschisis has an outer layer tear with a rolled posterior edge and an inner layer hole. Snail-track degeneration is found between 8:30 and 9:30. A meridional fold is seen at 4:30 with small tears at the posterior and inferior margins. There are atrophic retinal holes at 4:30 and a small localized retinal detachment is associated with holes at 5:30. Horseshoe retinal tears along with an operculated tear are seen between 6:30 and 8 o'clock. Note the pigment clump on the flap of the horseshoe tear at 6:30 and the vitreous strand on the flap of the tear at 7 o'clock. Peripheral cystoid degeneration is seen circumferentially next to the ora serrata. Courtesy of Matthew Garston and Anthony Cavallerano, Review of Optometry 1979;116:81–84.

3 Developmental Anomalies, Degenerations, and Diseases of the Peripheral Retina and Pars Plana

Pars Plana Cysts
and Epithelial Degeneration

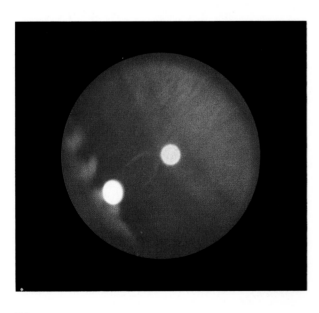

CLINICAL DESCRIPTION

Pars plana cysts are clear cystoid spaces between the pigmented and nonpigmented epithelia. Most large cysts are oval (Figures 3.1 and 3.2), but smaller ones can be round, oblong, lobulated, oval, or irregularly shaped. They vary in size from ¼ to 3 disc diameters and are usually located in the temporal side of the eye. Large cysts may occupy more than one bay and may extend from the ora serrata to the ciliary processes.

Figure 3.1 A pars plana cyst can be seen as an oval transparent ballooning (located between the light reflexes) on the superior nasal pars plana in a patient with posttraumatic aniridia. Also in view are the ciliary processes, the ora serrata, and the peripheral retina, seen through an indirect condensing lens.

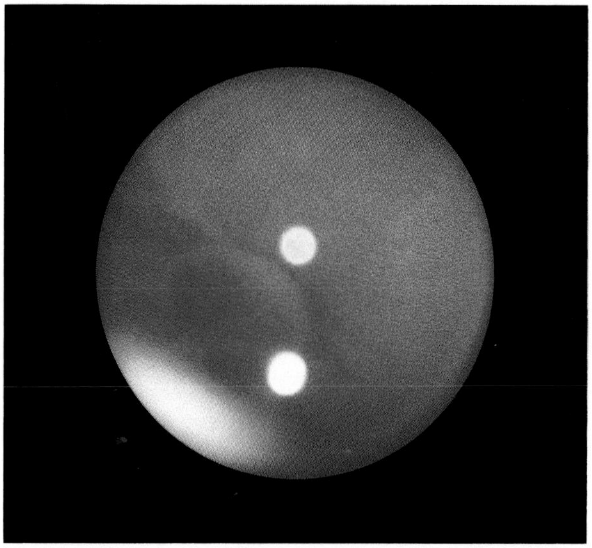

Figure 3.2 A roundish pars plana cyst is visible in an aphakic eye. The view is through an indirect condensing lens.

The inner walls may be flabby and poorly transparent or distended and very transparent. Most pars plana cysts exhibit a smooth, taut, transparent surface that allows a view of the underlying pigment epithelium. They may be solitary or occur in a row of multiple cysts abutting each other. Sometimes they have a light dusting of pigment on their inner walls. Pars plana cysts are present in 3% to 18% of all patients.[1-3]

HISTOPATHOLOGY

Pars plana cysts are formed by a separation of the nonpigmented from the pigmented epi-

Figure 3.3 The pars plana cyst consists of a separation of the nonpigmented epithelium from the pigmented epithelium of the pars plana by a fluid-filled cavity.

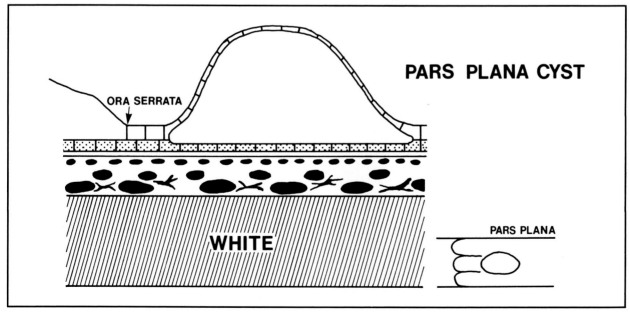

PARS PLANA CYST

ORA SERRATA

WHITE

PARS PLANA

thelium, which is analogous to a retinal detachment (Figure 3.3). The inner nonpigmented epithelium can be a single layer or consist of several cell layers.[2] The inner layer may even produce extensions into the cystic cavity.[4] The cavities are filled with a fluid which presumably contains hyaluronic acid.

CLINICAL SIGNIFICANCE

Most pars plana cysts are acquired and very few are congenital. They may be ideopathic or occur secondary to ocular disease. They are more commonly seen in eyes with retinal detachment, where they tend to be large in size. Their occurrence in eyes with retinal detachment may be the result of traction by the shrinking vitreous base.[5] The cysts may even communicate with the subretinal space in some cases. Pars plana cysts also frequently occur in eyes with posterior uveitis.

Pars plana cysts can be present in patients with multiple myeloma and seem to be filled with a para-aminosalicylic acid (PAS)-positive protein, which is the same myeloma protein (IgG) as found in the patients' serum.[6] During fixation, the cysts of multiple myeloma become whitish, whereas other pars plana cysts remain clear.[7]

The nonpigmented epithelium may show hyaline or fatty degeneration with increasing age. Hyperplasia of the nonpigmented epithelium may cause pedunculated or senile wartlike growths to appear.[4] There can be erosion of the nonpigmented epithelium, causing a craterlike appearance to the pars plana (Figure 3.4). Also, tears of the nonpigmented epithelium can oc-

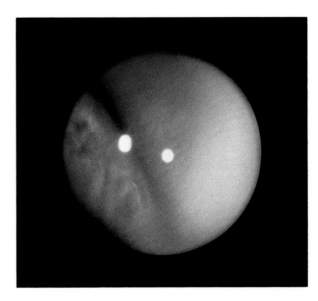

Figure 3.4 Degeneration of the superior temporal pars plana can be seen as areas of epithelial erosion, as viewed through the indirect condensing lens with scleral depression.

cur. These are usually found along the anterior margin of the vitreous base and they are generally associated with trauma.[5]

REFERENCES

1. Allen RA, Miller DH, et al. Cysts of the posterior ciliary body (pars plana). Arch Ophthalmol 1961;66:302–313.
2. Okun E. Gross and microscopic pathology in autopsy eyes. IV. Pars plana cysts. Am J Ophthalmol 1961;51:1221–1228.
3. Grignolo A, Schepens CL, et al. Cysts of the pars plana ciliaris. Arch Ophthalmol 1957;58:530–543.
4. Duke-Elder S, Perkins ES. Diseases of the uveal tract. In: System of ophthalmology, vol. 9. London: Henry Kimpton, 1977:765–768.
5. Schepens CL. Retinal detachment and allied diseases. Philadelphia: WB Saunders, 1983:163–187.
6. Bloch RS: Hematologic disorders. In: Duane TD, Jaeger EA, eds. Clinical ophthalmology, vol. 5. Philadelphia: Harper & Row, 1976:8.
7. Yanoff M, Fine BS. Ocular pathology: a text and atlas, ed. 2. Philadelphia: Harper & Row, 1982:404.

Retinal Pigment Epithelium Hypertrophy and Hyperplasia

Congenital hypertrophy or hyperplasia of the pigment epithelium is a benign and nonprogressive condition.

CLINICAL DESCRIPTION

Lesions are pigmented, flat, and round, with distinct margins (Figure 3.5). These areas are not to be confused with a choroidal nevus, which is usually flat, slate gray in color, and with indistinct margins. On rare occasions, the congenital hypertrophy has been shown to enlarge. It is not uncommon to observe a full or partial hypopigmented ring around the lesions (Figure 3.6), which is considered pathognomonic and is responsible for the term "haloed nevus" of the pigment epithelium.

Areas of hypertrophy or hyperplasia range in color from light brown to jet black, depending on the amount of melanin in the epithelial cells.[1]

Figure 3.5 Retinal pigment epithelium hypertrophy that is darkly pigmented.

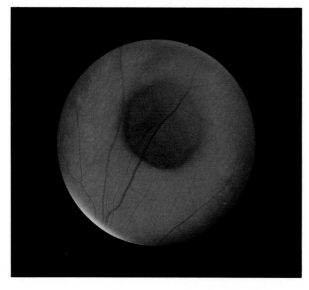

They can vary in size from a fraction of a disc diameter to several disc diameters. A number of smaller lesions aggregated in a localized area of the fundus is known as grouped pigmentation spots or "bear tracks" (Figure 3.7).[2] They are unilateral in about 85% of cases.[3]

Acquired hyperplasia of the pigment epithelium displays the same characteristics as the congenital form, except that lesions tend to be irregular in shape and do not have depigmented rings associated with them (see Pigment Clumping, page 39).

Areas of pigment mottling and chorioretinal atrophy often occur in the congenital form of these lesions (Figure 3.8). These windowlike areas of chorioretinal atrophy are known as lacunae and they allow a clear view of the underlying choroid (Figure 3.9). There may be a single lacuna or many lacunae present in an area of pigment epithelial hyperplasia (see Chorioretinal Atrophy, page 72).

There is some debate as to whether the congenital lesions are produced by hypertrophy (increased size of the pigment epithelial cells)[2,4] or by hyperplasia (increase in the number of epithelial cells).[5] It may well be that both processes can occur. Hyperplasia is probably the primary cause of the acquired lesions.

HISTOPATHOLOGY

There is either a hypertrophy or a hyperplasia present and the cells contain melanin granules that are larger than normal (Figure 3.10). This gives the lesions their darkly pigmented appearance. Above the lesions there is loss of photoreceptors, which explains why visual field defects can be plotted over these lesions.[3]

The lacunae seen in these lesions are the result of chorioretinal atrophy (Figure 3.9); an explanation of this process is covered under the heading of Chorioretinal Atrophy (see page 72).

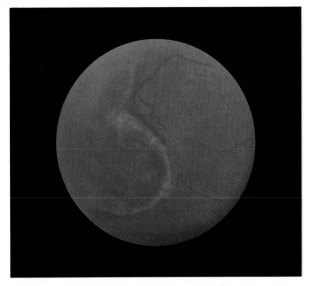

Figure 3.6 Retinal pigment epithelium hypertrophy that is moderately pigmented and has a classic clear halo around it.

Figure 3.7 Grouped pigmentation spots or "bear tracks" are the result of hyperplasia or hypertrophy of the retinal pigment epithelium.

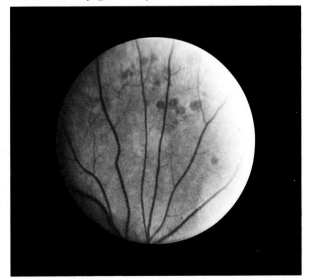

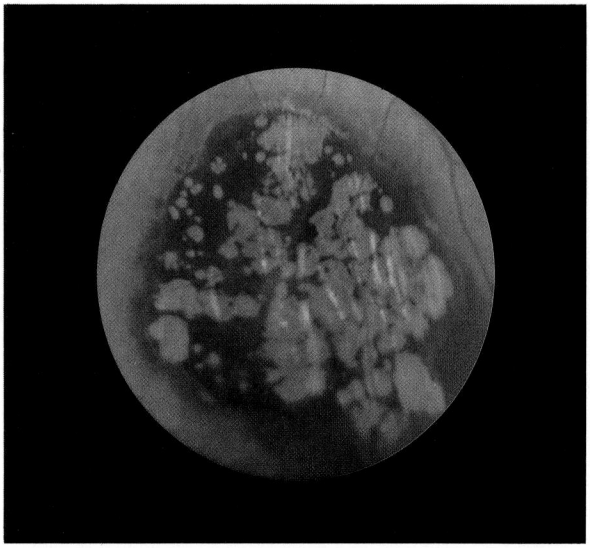

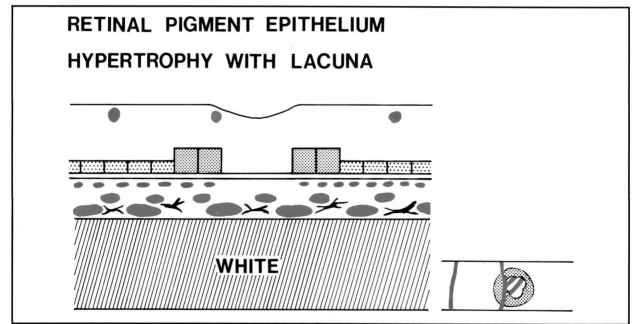

Figure 3.8 Retinal pigment epithelial hypertrophy with numerous lacunae (chorioretinal atrophy) and a slight clear halo around it.

CLINICAL SIGNIFICANCE

The congenital lesions are benign but present a diagnostic challenge for the clinician, since the differential diagnosis includes choroidal nevi and melanomas. The acquired form is the result of some type of stimulus to the pigment epithelium and may denote a past episode of trauma or other postinflammatory or degenerative process. The acquired lesions are less of a diagnostic problem because of their irregular appearance. Pigment clumps can be associated with vitreous traction and retinal breaks.

Figure 3.9 Note that chorioretinal atrophy has resulted in the formation of a lacuna within the lesion.

RETINAL PIGMENT EPITHELIUM HYPERTROPHY WITH LACUNA

WHITE

REFERENCES

1. Purcell JJ, Shields JA. Hypertrophy with hyperpigmentation of the retinal pigment epithelium. Arch Ophthalmol 1975;93:1122–1126.
2. Shields JA, Tso MO. Congenital grouped pigmentation of the retina. Arch Ophthalmol 1975; 93:1153–1156.
3. Yanoff M, Fine BS. Ocular pathology: a text and atlas, ed 2. Philadelphia: Harper & Row, 1982:476–814.
4. Buettner H. Congenital hypertrophy of the pigment epithelium. Am J Ophthalmol 1975; 79:177–189.
5. Hogan MJ, Zimmerman LE. Ophthalmic pathology: an atlas and textbook, ed. 2. Philadelphia: WB Saunders, 1962:436.

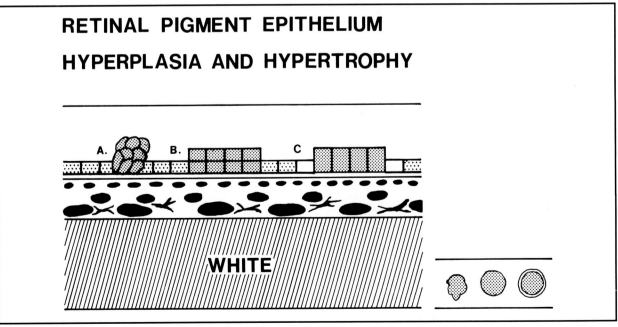

Figure 3.10 (A) Hypertrophy of the pigment epithelium that is most likely acquired from an inflammatory stimulus and developed an irregular shape. (B) A congenital hyperplasia with its more uniform and round shape. (C) Congenital hypertrophy of the pigment epithelium with a clear halo resulting from the absence of melanin in the pigment epithelial cells adjacent to the lesion.

Choroidal Nevus

Figure 3.11 Choroidal nevus. Note the slate gray color, indistinct margins, and flat appearance.

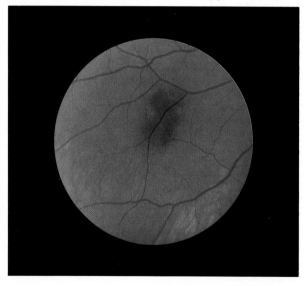

CLINICAL DESCRIPTION

A choroidal nevus, which is a pigmented area of the fundus, can have a varied appearance. Nevi usually vary in size from a fraction of a disc diameter to many disc diameters. There are some cases in which they can be as large as half of the fundus and rarely they can involve the entire fundus.[1] Nevi are usually flat but they can be elevated from one to two diopters.

Choroidal nevi appear slate gray in color (Figure 3.11), which may be the result of viewing them through the pigment epithelium. They have indistinct margins due to random gathering of melanocytes at the margins of the nevus. Also, viewing the edges of the nevus through the pigment epithelium tends to haze the margins. Amelanotic nevi are the result of melanocytes that are not capable of producing melanin.

Choroidal nevi can have a mottled coloration that is secondary to degeneration of the overlying pigment epithelium and formation of drusen. Visual field defects can sometimes be plotted over these lesions, and they may rarely hyperfluoresce during fluorescein angiography. Choroidal nevi usually produce hypofluorescent areas during fluorescein angiography. Ciliary body or choroidal nevi are found in at least 30% of people.[1]

HISTOPATHOLOGY

A choroidal nevus is a benign accumulation of melanocytes (tumor) within the choroid (Figure 3.12). Nevi appear as flat lesions within the choroid, displaying variable degrees of pigmentation. Cell-types of this lesion vary from a polygonal plump shape to elongated spindle shape with branching processes. These cells are arranged in compact layers and generally the thicker the nevus, the more darkly pigmented they look. Many times there is loss of photoreceptors in the retina above the lesions.

Figure 3.12 The choroidal nevus is composed of an aggregation of melanocytes within the choroid.

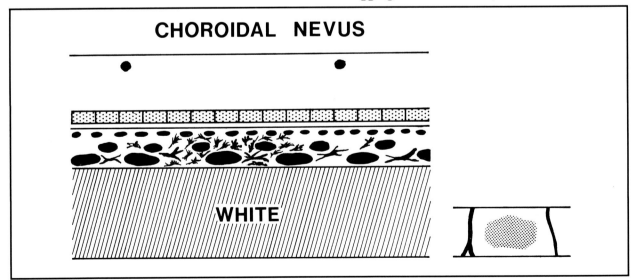

CLINICAL SIGNIFICANCE

The main clinical significance of a choroidal nevus lies in distinguishing it from a choroidal melanoma.[2-4] Many authorities believe that choroidal nevi have the potential to transform into melanoma. Therefore they should be followed on a periodic basis with either drawings or fundus photographs. Any documented growth of a nevus should be suspected as a potentially malignant sign, especially if the lesion is five disc diameters or greater in size.

REFERENCES

1. Yanoff M, Fine BS. Ocular pathology: a text and atlas, ed. 2. Philadelphia: Harper & Row, 1982:788, 826, 831.
2. Gass JDM. Problems in the differential diagnosis of choroidal nevi and malignant melanomas. Am J Ophthalmol 1977;83:299–323.
3. Zimmerman LE. Problems in the diagnosis of malignant melanomas of the choroid and ciliary body. Am J Ophthalmol 1970;75:917–929.
4. Shields JA, McDonald PR. Improvements in the diagnosis of posterior uveal melanoma. Arch Ophthalmol 1974;91:259–264.

Malignant Choroidal Melanoma

A melanoma, although rare, is the most frequently occurring malignant intraocular tumor in adults. Incidence in the white population over the age of 50 years is 21 per million per year.[1] The tumor is usually a mottled, elevated mass in the fundus and often has a brown to greenish gray color.[2-4] The mottled appearance is the result of drusen and degeneration of the pigment epithelium above the tumor. It is not uncommon to find orange stipples on the surface of this tumor (Figure 3.13) as the result of accumulation of lipofuscin (a wear-and-tear pigment released from the degenerating pigment epithelial cells).[5,6]

CLINICAL DESCRIPTION

The tumor may be flat and diffuse, but commonly it is an elevated, rounded mass. The elevation may only be a few millimeters or the

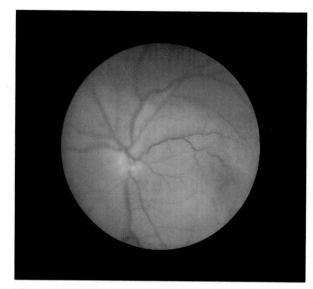

Figure 3.13   A juxtapapillary melanoma of the choroid is shown because of its characteristic physical findings. Note the circular hazy area in the inferior central portion of the tumor. This is a small serous retinal detachment. Also note the golden orange-colored spots on the surface of the tumor, which denote areas of concentrated lipofuscin. Tumor elevation is detected by observing the blood vessels traversing upward onto the tumor.

mass may completely fill the vitreous cavity. The tumor is usually a rounded mass without lobular extensions when it is contained beneath the basal lamina (Bruch's membrane); however, it often takes on a so-called collar-button appearance after breaking through the basal lamina.

The size can vary from a few millimeters in diameter, generally from about 5 to 7, to a lesion that occupies a majority of the fundus. Most malignant melanomas range from 10 to 20 mm in diameter when initially discovered. The rate of growth of a choroidal melanoma is typically slow, and over extended periods of time there may be no growth observed; however, there have been cases in which rapid growth was observed in only 60 days.[7]

Many melanomas have an associated secondary nonrhegmatogenous retinal detachment, which can be shifting in nature. This type of retinal detachment is seen in about 2% of eyes with a choroidal melanoma.[8] The detachment can be small and localized to the surface of the tumor (Figures 3.13 and 3.14) or it may be extensive and found some distance from the tumor. The secondary detachment is composed of a serous fluid that is somewhat viscous and tends to shift positions due to gravity.[9,10] Thus the tumor may be located in the superior half of the ocular fundus, but the detachment is often located in the inferior dependent region when the patient is examined in the sitting position. When the patient reclines, the detachment is relocated in the posterior pole of the fundus. The serous detachment associated with a choroidal tumor typically does not extend to the ora serrata. Often, loss of vision due to retinal detachment is the presenting symptom of a melanoma of the choroid. Sometimes the tumor is hidden by the retinal detachment, and shifting the patient's position during the examination may uncover its existence. A break that forms in a serous retinal detachment can confuse the diagnosis by making the clinician believe it is a primary rhegmatogenous retinal detachment. Other ocular complications associated with an intraocular melanoma include uveitis and glaucoma.

Any suspected tumor of the ocular fundus should be followed with serial fundus drawings or photographs to document changes in its physical characteristics. A documented change in size necessitates referral to a retinal specialist.

HISTOPATHOLOGY

The tumor is composed of malignant melanocytes, which are either spindle or epithelioid in shape. Sometimes the cell type cannot be determined due to tumor necrosis. The epithelioid cell has a much higher degree of malignancy associated with it and thus a higher frequency of patient fatality. The tumor may not

Figure 3.14 Histopathologic section of the eye in Figure 3.13 showing juxtapapillary malignant melanoma that gives no sign of invading the optic nerve (small arrow). The dimensions of the tumor were 9 × 5 × 3 mm. Note the serous retinal detachment on the surface of the tumor, with fluid visible beneath the large arrow, underneath the detachment. Other sites of retinal detachment are the result of histologic preparation and thus display no evidence of serous fluid. The large arrow points to a retinal break that resulted from the histologic preparation.

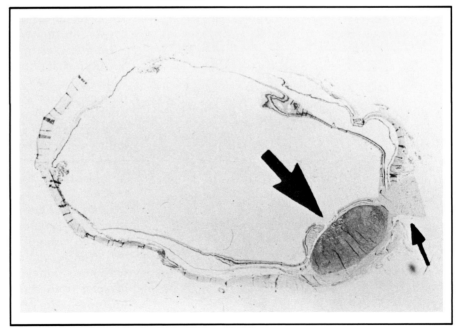

be homogeneous in cell type, and it is not unusual to find epithelioid cells in the center that are surrounded by spindle cells. The tumor is seen as a pigmented mass within the choroid (Figure 3.14) in the early stage, but later it may break through the basal lamina (Bruch's membrane) or penetrate the sclera in more advanced stages.

CLINICAL SIGNIFICANCE

The significance of a melanoma of the choroid is its potential for fatal consequences. The primary intraocular tumor usually spreads by way of the circulatory system to the liver. The patient dies secondary to liver failure. The other two most common sites of metastasis are the lungs and brain. A metastatic work-up is necessary for all patients diagnosed with an intraocular melanoma; this consists of liver function studies, liver, lung, and brain, scans and chest x-ray.

The conventional treatment for intraocular choroidal melanoma has been enucleation.[11] After analyses of melanoma data, however, it is apparent that enucleation may not prevent death from metastasis and may in fact contribute to increased mortality by spread of the tumor at the time of surgery.[12,13] For that reason, authorities have increasingly relied on specialized modalities of irradiation for melanomas, including charged-particle irradiation with proton beams or helium nuclei.[14-16] Radioactive episcleral plaques sutured over the melanoma have also proved successful.[17] Less common forms of treatment include photocoagulation, cryotherapy, and chemotherapy.[11,18]

Yearly metastatic evaluation of patients with known melanomas has been recommended because of the tendency for metastases to show up months to years after treatment or enucleation.

REFERENCES

1. Yanoff M, Fine BS. Ocular pathology: a text and atlas, ed. 2. Philadelphia: Harper & Row, 1982:788, 826, 831.

2. Reese AB. Tumors of the eye, ed. 3. Hagerstown, MD: Harper & Row, 1976.

3. Gass JDM. Differential diagnosis of intraocular tumors. A stereoscopic presentation. St. Louis: CV Mosby, 1974.

4. Jacobiec FA. Ocular and adnexal tumors. Birmingham, AL: Aesculapius, 1978.

5. Shields JA, Rodrigues MM, et al. Lipofuscin pigment over benign and malignant choroidal tumors. Trans Am Acad Ophthalmol Otolaryngol 1976;81:871–881.

6. Font RL, Zimmerman LE, et al. The nature of the orange pigment over a choroidal melanoma: histochemical and electron microscopal observations. Arch Ophthalmol 1974;91:359–362.

7. Friberg TR, Fineberg E, et al. Extremely rapid growth of a primary choroidal melanoma. Arch Ophthalmol 1983;101:1375–1377.

8. Boniuk M, Zimmerman LE. Occurrence and behavior of choroidal melanomas in eyes subjected to operations for retinal detachment. Trans Am Acad Ophthalmol Otolaryngol 1962;66:642–657.

9. Pischel DK. Retinal detachment: a manual, ed. 2. Am Acad Ophthalmol Otolaryngol 1965:80–81.

10. Schepens CL. Retinal detachment and allied diseases. Philadelphia: Harper & Row, 1983: 224–225, 705–730.

11. Shields JA. Current approaches to the diagnosis and management of choroidal melanomas. Surv Ophthalmol 1977;21:443–463.

12. Zimmerman LE, McLean IW. An evaluation of enucleation in the management of uveal melanoma. Am J Ophthalmol 1979;87:741–760.

13. Zimmerman LE, McLean IW. Metastatic disease from untreated uveal melanoma. Am J Ophthalmol 1979;88:524–534.

14. Gragoudas ES, Goitein M, et al. Proton beam irradiation of uveal melanoma. Arch Ophthalmol 1982;100:928–934.

15. Char DH, Phillips TD. The potential for adjunct

radiation radiotherapy in choroidal melanoma. Arch Ophthalmol 1982;100:247–248.

16. Char DH, Castro JR. Helium ion therapy for choroidal melanoma. Arch Ophthalmol 1982; 100:935–938.

17. Packer S, Rotman M, et al. Irradiation of choroidal melanoma with iodine 125 ophthalmic plaque. Arch Ophthalmol 1980;98:1453–1457.

18. Minckler D, Thompson FB. Photocoagulation of malignant melanoma. Arch Ophthalmol 1979;97:120–123.

Pigment Clumping

CLINICAL DESCRIPTION

Pigment clumps are small areas of increased pigmentation of the retina, usually less than one disc diameter in size (Figure 3.15). The clumps may invade the retina and result in a slight elevation of the involved retina. These lesions are generally located in the equatorial region of the retina, rarely posterior to the equator. They seem to occur in all quadrants of the fundus without predilection for a particular one.

HISTOPATHOLOGY

Pigment clumps are the result of benign proliferation of pigment epithelial cells into the retina (Figure 3.10A). This may be a developmental condition or be acquired secondary to traction or localized irritation.

Figure 3.15 Pigment clump with a small adjacent area of chorioretinal atrophy and attachment of a vitreous band (arrow). The view is through an indirect condensing lens.

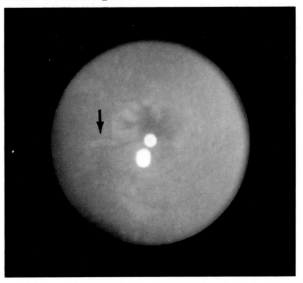

CLINICAL SIGNIFICANCE

It is not uncommon to find vitreous traction in areas of pigment clumping. The clumps may have a small retinal break associated with them or exhibit a surrounding ring of white-with-pressure.[1] A retinal flap from a tear may have as associated pigment clump (see Figure 2.10, page 19). Clumps in the equatorial region are more likely to produce a retinal break than those found close to the ora serrata.[2]

REFERENCES

1. Dumas J, Schepens CL. Chorioretinal lesions predisposing to retinal breaks. Am J Ophthalmol 1966;61:620–630.
2. Schepens CL. Retinal detachment and allied diseases. Philadelphia: WB Saunders, 1983:164.

Peripheral Senile
Pigmentary Degeneration

CLINICAL DESCRIPTION

Peripheral senile pigmentary degeneration (also known as peripheral tapetochoroidal degeneration) gives a pigmented, granular appearance to the peripheral retina and is usually found between the ora serrata and the equator. Areas of hyperpigmentation and hypopigmentation scatter in a circumferential band. The anterior border is irregular and difficult to see, but the posterior border is smooth and well defined.[1] When the pigmentation takes on the appearance of a fine network, it is called reticular pigmentary degeneration (Figure 3.16).

This entity does not cause defects on visual fields or dark-adaptation studies. It commonly occurs in persons over 40 years of age, reportedly in 20% of this population. It is bilateral in almost every case.[2]

Figure 3.16 Reticular senile peripheral retinal pigmentary degeneration seen through the indirect condensing lens. Note crisscrossing pattern to the lines of pigmentation.

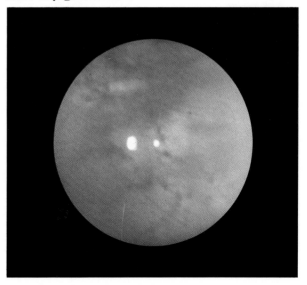

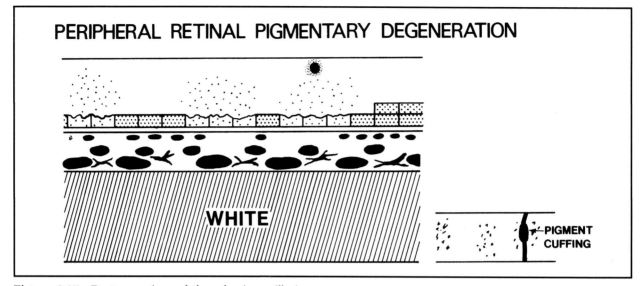

Figure 3.17 Degeneration of the choriocapillaris and pigment epithelium leads to dispersion of pigment granules in the sensory retina. Macrophages may engulf the melanin granules and carry them into the retina, where they may deposit the granules along venules (pigment cuffing) during diapedesis.

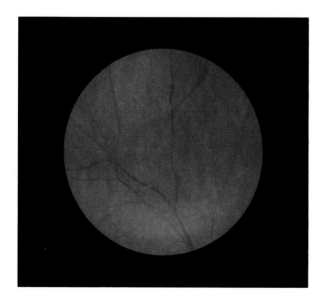

HISTOPATHOLOGY

The pigment epithelium displays some cells with loss of pigment granules and others with an increase in pigment granules (Figure 3.17). Pigment released from degenerating pigment epithelial cells is scattered in the retinal tissue. There is also some loss of photoreceptors, thickening of the basal lamina, and arteriosclerosis of the choriocapillaris. Macrophages may engulf the melanin granules and carry them to the retinal venules, where they may deposit the granules along the venules (pigment cuffing) during diapedesis (Figures 3.17 and 3.18).

Figure 3.18 Two areas of pigment cuffing along retinal venules.

CLINICAL SIGNIFICANCE

This is an involutionary process and does not require treatment. Confusion may exist over the possibility of retinitis pigmentosa; the pigmentation in this condition usually has a bone-spicule appearance, but sometimes it may be granular. Other signs necessary to diagnose retinitis pigmentosa are a waxy yellow pallor to the disc, visual field defects, attenuated vessels, night blindness, and an abnormal electroretinogram.

REFERENCES

1. Foos RY, Spencer LM, et al. Trophic degeneration of the peripheral retina. In: New Orleans Academy of Ophthalmology: symposium on retina and retinal surgery. St. Louis: CV Mosby, 1969.
2. Straatsma BR, Foos RY, et al. Degenerative diseases of the peripheral retina. In: Duane TD, Jaeger EA, eds. Clinical ophthalmology, vol. 3. Philadelphia: Harper & Row, 1980;26:8–10.

Peripheral Chorioretinal Degeneration

Figure 3.19 Peripheral chorioretinal degeneration is seen as a whitish band just posterior to the ora serrata. View is of the nasal ora serrata through the indirect condensing lens with scleral depression.

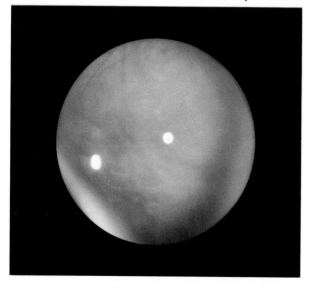

CLINICAL DESCRIPTION

Peripheral chorioretinal degeneration is a whitish smooth area adjacent to the ora serrata (Figure 3.19). The posterior edge merges discretely into the normal retina without producing an obvious demarcation line. The pigment epithelium under the chorioretinal degeneration is hyperpigmented.

This degeneration usually does not extend more than two disc diameters from the ora serrata. Blood vessels that pass through an area of chorioretinal degeneration may become sclerotic and may be surrounded by pigment. The more advanced areas of degeneration occur closer to the ora serrata, perhaps as the result of irritation of the peripheral retina by traction forces on the vitreous base.[1]

Peripheral chorioretinal degeneration is found in about two-thirds of the population to some degree. It generally begins in the fourth decade of life and increases with age.[2] There appears to be no predilection either for sex or for location in the peripheral fundus.

HISTOPATHOLOGY

Chorioretinal degeneration is highlighted by decreased profusion of the peripheral retinal and choroidal blood vessels (Figure 3.20). This is probably the result of arteriosclerosis. There is degeneration and shrinkage of the retinal tissue and subsequent glial proliferation. The atrophic retina becomes tightly adherent to the underlying choroid. Because this is a fairly mild degenerative process, there is gliotic repair and reactive pigment proliferation. If this process is severe, repair is not possible and chorioretinal atrophy will result.[2]

CLINICAL SIGNIFICANCE

Peripheral chorioretinal degeneration and peripheral cystoid degeneration commonly occur in the same region of the fundus and have

Figure 3.20 Note the loss of the choriocapillaris and the retinal degeneration located posterior to the ora serrata.

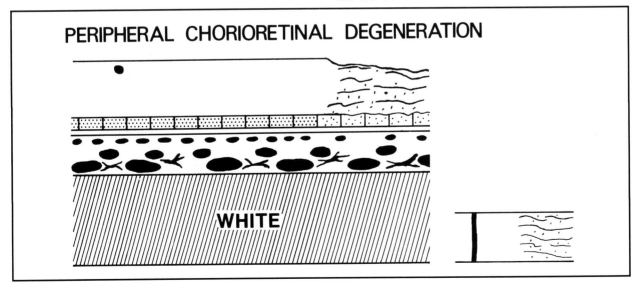

PERIPHERAL CHORIORETINAL DEGENERATION

WHITE

many of the same degenerative characteristics. These two conditions seem to inhibit each other, as chorioretinal degeneration is frequently found posterior to cystoid degeneration and acts as a natural barrier to the posterior progression of cystoid degeneration.[2] Peripheral chorioretinal degeneration appears to be benign and does not seem to play a role in the production of retinal breaks.

REFERENCES

1. Goldbaum MH. Retinal examination and surgery. In: Peyman GA, Sanders DR, Goldberg MF, eds. Principles and practice of ophthalmology, vol. 2. Philadelphia: WB Saunders, 1980; 15:1029.
2. Schepens CL. Retinal detachment and allied diseases. Philadelphia: WB Saunders, 1983:145–154.

Peripheral Retinal Hemorrhage

CLINICAL DESCRIPTION

Peripheral retinal hemorrhages appear as red spots that are usually less than one disc diameter in size (frequently ⅛ to ¼ mm). Hemorrhages located in the peripheral retina are of various shapes but they are usually irregularly round or oval (Figure 3.21). Unlike a hemorrhage, retinal holes are almost always symmetrically round. The overlying retina is flat, and upon depressing these small peripheral hemorrhages, they roll smoothly, without exhibiting an edge as is seen when rolling a hole (see Figures 3.53 and 3.54). Flame-shaped hemorrhages are found in the superficial retinal layers and derive their shape from their characteristic orientation in the nerve fiber layer. Most peripheral hemorrhages are blot- and dot-shaped and are found in the middle layers of the retina. Small peripheral hemorrhages tend to be absorbed rather quickly but at times they can take several months to absorb.

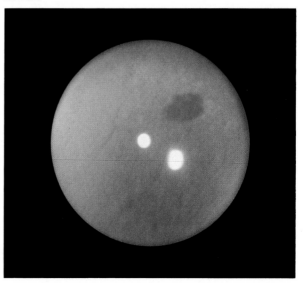

Figure 3.21   A peripheral retinal hemorrhage seen through the indirect condensing lens. Note that there is no degenerated or detached retinal tissue around the hemorrhages, as might be found with a retinal break.

47

HISTOPATHOLOGY

Most of these hemorrhages result from a bleed in the deep capillary bed of the retina. They may be the result of a localized degeneration in the vessel wall or be produced by an increase in venous pressure. It is far more common to have a bleed in the venous system than in the arterial system of the retina.

CLINICAL SIGNIFICANCE

Peripheral retinal hemorrhages can be secondary to any type of hemorrhagic retinopathy, for example, diabetes, hypertension, blood dyscrasias, etc. They also commonly occur in venous stasis conditions and not infrequently seen in patients with chronic obstructive pulmonary disease (COPD).[1] Finally, they are often ideopathic or secondary to old age. These hemorrhages usually resolve without any sequelae and it may be impossible to detect their previous retinal location.

A retinal hemorrhage that is mostly round can be mistaken for a retinal hole. A discussion on the differential diagnosis of a small round retinal hemorrhage and a retinal hole can be found in Chapter 5, page 153.

REFERENCE

1.   Gottlieb, F, Harris D, et al. The peripheral eyeground in chronic respiratory disease. Arch Ophthalmol 1969;82:611–619.

Peripheral Retinal Neovascularization

Peripheral retinal neovascularization occurs in a number of ocular disease conditions and from iatrogenic causes. Neovascularization of the near retinal periphery is most commonly seen in proliferative diabetic retinopathy.

CLINICAL DESCRIPTION

In the far periphery of the retina, the most common cause of neovascularization appears to be related to sickle cell retinopathy. It characteristically displays a proliferative vascular formation known as a sea fan, which resembles the marine invertebrate *Gorgonia flabellum*. Fibrosis and intraretinal and preretinal hemorrhages are often associated with sea fans. Sometimes a vitreous detachment may elevate the sea fan into the vitreous cavity. Sea fans are seen in 59% to 72% of patients with the SC form of the disease,[1,2] in 33% of patients with sickle cell-thal-

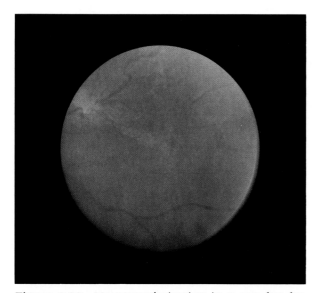

Figure 3.22 Neovascularization in a sea fan formation can be seen in the temporal periphery just distal to the site of an old peripheral branch vein occlusion. Note the retinal fibrosis at the site of the original occlusion.

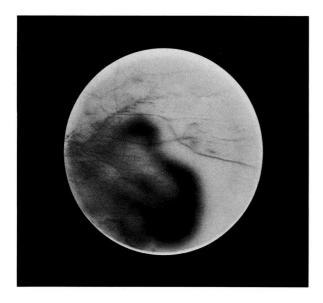

assemia,[3] and uncommonly in patients with the other hemoglobinopathies (10%).[1]

Sea fans are most frequently located in the superior temporal quadrant and, in descending order of frequency, the inferior temporal, superior nasal, and inferior nasal quadrants.[4] They may grow in a circumferential pattern and rarely do they come close to the posterior pole. Other retinal findings include so-called salmon patches and black sunbursts.

Retrolental fibroplasia can also produce neovascularization of the far retinal periphery. Less commonly it occurs during the recovery phase of branch vein occlusions[5] (Figures 3.22 and 3.23) and after incisions into the vitreous through the pars plana and peripheral retina during retinal and vitreous surgery.[6]

HISTOPATHOLOGY

Trypsin-digest studies of sickle cell retinopathy show arteriolar occlusions, peripheral zones of infarcted capillaries, arteriovenous anastomoses, capillary budding microaneurysmal formations, vessel enlargement, and neovascular tissue. Sometimes vitreous traction bands are attached to the neovascular tissue.[4]

The neovascular tissue demonstrates marked endothelial proliferation arising from residual vascular complexes immediately adjacent to areas of retinal capillary closure.

Figure 3.23 Fluorescein angiography of the neovascular area in Figure 3.22, 116 seconds post injection. Note the massive profusion of the dye from the neovascular tissue.

CLINICAL SIGNIFICANCE

Hemorrhaging is the all too common consequence of neovascularization anywhere in the eye. Vitreous hemorrhage is a fairly common event in peripheral retinal neovascularization and was present in 23% of patients with SC sickle cell disease and 3% of patients with the SS trait.[3]

After a vitreous hemorrhage there is vitreous degeneration and scarring, which frequently lead to increased vitreous traction on the retina. The traction may result in a retinal break and subsequent rhegmatogenous retinal detachment.[7] Sometimes with severe vitreous traction, a tractional retinal detachment may be produced.

Treatment for peripheral neovascularization of the retina consists of one or a combination of the following modalities: photocoagulation, diathermy, and transconjunctival cryotherapy.[8-10]

REFERENCES

1. Welsh RB, Goldberg MF. Sickle-cell hemoglobin and its relation to fundus abnormalities. Arch Ophthalmol 1966;75:353–362.
2. Goldberg MF. Natural history of untreated proliferative sickle cell retinopathy. Am J Ophthalmol 1971;71:649–665.
3. Goldberg MF, Charache S, et al. Ophthalmologic manifestations of sickle cell thalassemia. Arch Intern Med 1971;128:33–39.
4. Goldberg MF. Sickle cell retinopathy. In: Duane TD, Jaeger EA, eds. Clinical ophthalmology, vol. 3. Philadelphia: Harper & Row, 1979;17:1–45.
5. Jaeger EA. Venous obstructive disease of the retina. In: Duane TD, Jaeger EA, eds. Clinical ophthalmology, vol. 3. Philadelphia: Harper & Row, 1979;15:1–21.
6. Schepens CL. Retinal detachment and allied diseases. Philadelphia: WB Saunders, 1983: 1042.

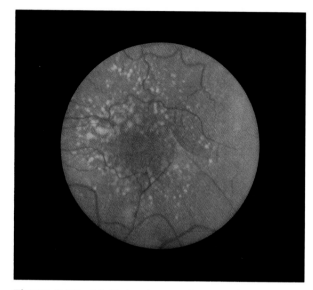

Figure 3.25 Multiple drusen in macula, some of which have coalesced into larger drusen bodies. Note the preretinal membrane just temporal to the fovea, which is peeling down on itself and appears curved on its superotemporal border.

Figure 3.26 Note that the drusen have elevated and thinned the pigment epithelium, which makes them appear rather transparent when seen through the retina.

This same phenomenon produces a window defect during fluorescein angiography that results in early hyperfluorescent spots during the choroidal flush and a gradual diminution as the concentration of fluorescein in the choroid decreases.

HISTOPATHOLOGY

Drusen are focal, irregular, homogeneous, moundlike extensions of the basal lamina (Bruch's membrane) (Figure 3.26). They are most likely the deposit of a hyaline material (an acid mucopolysaccharide) from degenerated pigment epithelial cells onto the cuticular portion of the basal lamina. Since drusen commonly occur with increasing age, natural degeneration of the choroidal vessels and pigment epithelium is probably responsible for most of them. The pigment epithelium appears degenerated and stretched thin over the drusen. Drusen can undergo further degeneration and the hyaline material may be replaced with dystrophic calcium, thus giving them a white appearance.[1]

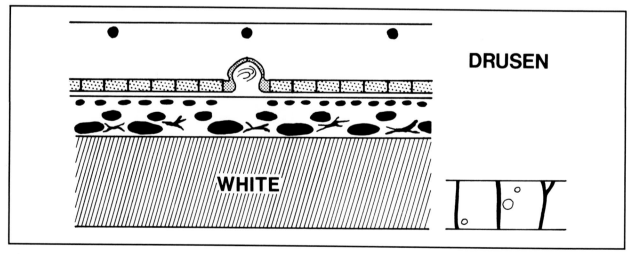

CLINICAL SIGNIFICANCE

Peripheral retinal drusen are generally considered a benign degeneration that increases with age and produces little consequence in most cases. Rarely, they are involved in the formation of a peripheral subretinal neovascular membrane.[2] They can be associated with a number of ocular and systemic diseases such as dysproteinemia, chronic leukemia, pseudoxanthoma elasticum, scleroderma, Rendu-Osler-Weber syndrome, and many other conditions.[3] It is not uncommon to find drusen overlying choroidal tumors, for example, malignant melanoma. They are seen in Doyne's honeycomb choroiditis, also known as dominant and familial drusen.

REFERENCES

1. Cavender JC, Ai E. Hereditary macular dystrophies. In: Duane TD, Jaeger EA, eds. Clinical ophthalmology, vol. 3. Philadelphia: Harper & Row, 1982;9:18–19.
2. Gass JDM. Drusen and disciform macular detachment and degeneration. Arch Ophthalmol 1973;90:206–217.
3. Duke-Elder S, Perkins ES. Diseases of the uveal tract. In: System of ophthalmology, vol. 10. London: Henry Kimpton, 1977;5:536.

Retinal Tufts

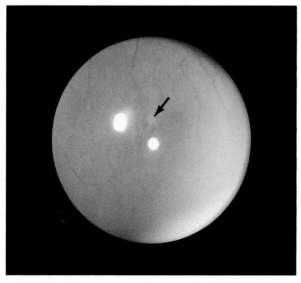

Figure 3.27 Peripheral retinal tuft (arrow) seen through the indirect condensing lens.

CLINICAL DESCRIPTION

Retinal tufts, also known as granular tissue, are grayish to white lesions in the peripheral retina that have a dull, irregular appearance (Figure 3.27). They are usually very small, ranging from a few microns to approximately 3 mm, and have a great variety of shapes. Zonular traction tufts vary from barely raised to markedly elevated.

These lesions may be solitary and isolated or occur in clusters (Figure 3.28). They are generally located between the equator and the ora serrata, commonly in the nasal half of the fundus.[1] The usual location is just posterior to the ora serrata within the vitreous base. These lesions seem to have a preference for the nasal half of the fundus and tend to occur bilaterally.[2,3] Vitreous traction is usually present and is frequently attached to the apex of the tuft. Vitreous traction may pull small pieces of the

Figure 3.28 Three peripheral retinal tufts seen in the indirect condensing lens with scleral depression.

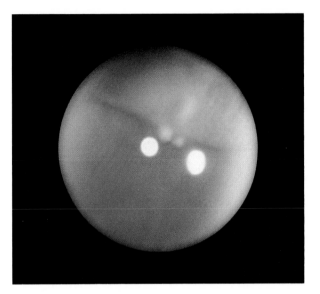

Figure 3.29 Cystic retinal tuft with vitreous traction.

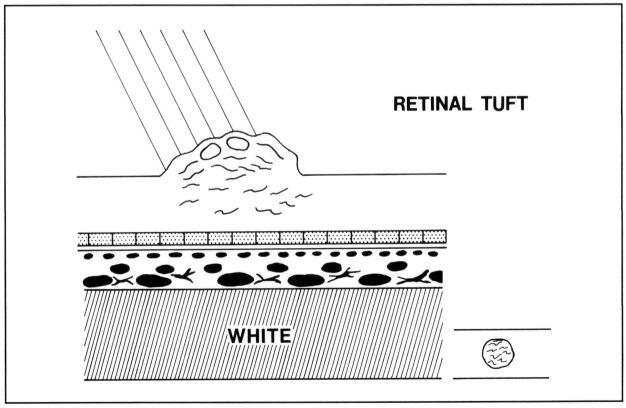

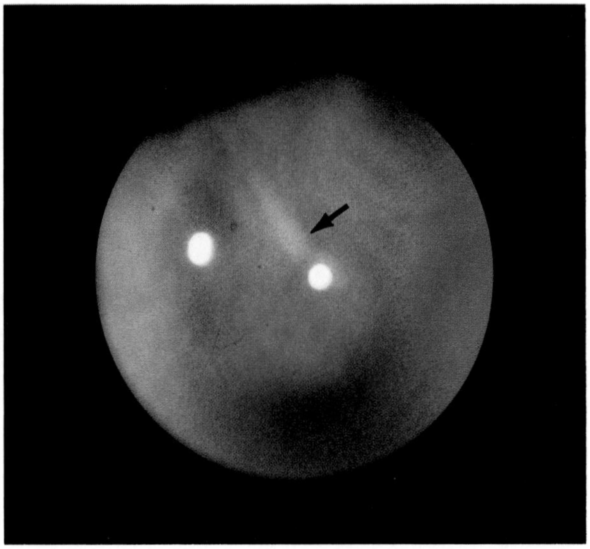

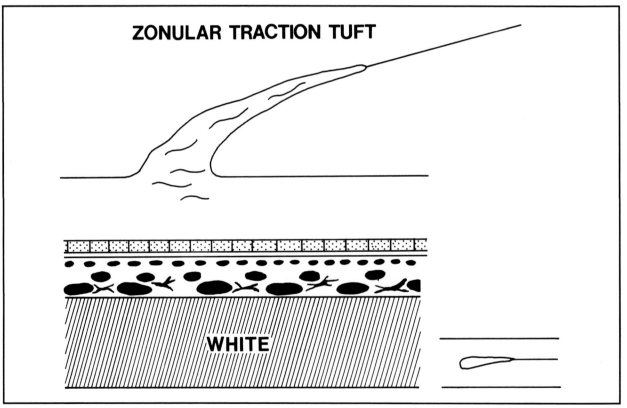

Figure 3.30 Zonular traction tuft seen through the indirect condensing lens. The retina is to the right and the pars plana is to the left.

Figure 3.31 Vitreous zonule is pulling the retinal tuft in an anterior direction.

ZONULAR TRACTION TUFT

WHITE

tuft into the vitreous, producing a small vitreous floater. These lesions remain stationary in size and do not increase in number with age, suggesting that they are developmental in origin.[4]

Retinal tufts have several clinical appearances. A noncystic retinal tuft is a noncystic retinal degeneration composed of degenerated retinal tissue and proliferated glial cells. They are most often located in the vitreous base and can be found in any quadrant of the fundus. Noncystic tufts tend to be small and irregularly shaped, and may have pointed projections on their surface. They are present in 72% of the adult population and occur bilaterally in half of the cases.[5]

A cystic retinal tuft is the result of cystic retinal degeneration, in which a number of microcystic spaces are found in the lesion (Figure 3.29). These tend to be larger than noncystic tufts and they have a more honeycombed appearance. They are found in 5% of the adult population and are bilateral in only 6% of cases.[5]

A zonular traction tuft is produced by the tractional force of a zonule. The developing inner layer of the optic cup may produce zonules posterior to the ora serrata,[6] and as the globe grows, a zonule attached to the peripheral retina may pull retinal tissue forward into a traction tuft. The appearance is that of gliotic tissue being pulled anteriorly into the vitreous, making a sharp angle with the retina (Figure 3.30). The length of these tufts varies greatly, probably as a result of the difference in tractional forces. They have a triangular base that thins to a fairly sharp point at the apex (Figure 3.31). These lesions occur in 15% of the population and are present bilaterally in 15% of cases.[6] They are commonly found in the nasal half of the fundus and usually their base is less than 0.5 mm from the ora serrata.[7]

Retinal or granular tags consist of degenerated tissue that has been thinned and elongated by vitreous traction. They tend to be very small and sometimes are just barely visible during indirect ophthalmoscopy. They usually appear as tiny white posts protruding from the retinal surface into the vitreous (Figures 2.3 and 3.33). It is not uncommon to find these lesions associated with other peripheral degenerative anomalies such as meridional folds. Vitreous traction can cause these tufts to be avulsed from the retinal surface, resulting in a vitreous floater or retinal break.

HISTOPATHOLOGY

Retinal tufts are composed of degenerated retinal tissue and proliferated glial cells. Retinal disorganization seems to involve the entire sensory retina and there can be an associated disruption of the pigment epithelium. Frequently, microcytic degeneration occurs and vitreous traction is almost always present (Figure 3.29).

CLINICAL SIGNIFICANCE

Vitreous traction is mainly responsible for the formation of the retinal breaks associated with retinal tufts. The continuous tractional forces can cause both retinal holes and tears. These breaks can occur on any side of a retinal tag, a noncystic tuft, or a cystic tuft; however, zonular traction tufts tend to form retinal breaks on the posterior edge of their base. Retinal tufts with breaks are watched or treated depending on the clinical circumstances. Treatment consists of either cryopexy or photocoagulation.

REFERENCES

1. Teng CC, Katzin HM. An anatomic study of the periphery of the retina. Part 1. Nonpigmented epithelial cell proliferation and hole formation. Am J Ophthalmol 1951;34:1237–1248.

2. Spencer LM, Foos RY. Paravascular vitreoretinal attachments. Arch Ophthalmol 1970; 84:557–564.

3. Spencer LM, Straatsma BR, et al. Tractional degenerations of the peripheral retina. In: New Orleans Academy of Ophthalmology: symposium on retina and retinal surgery. St. Louis: CV Mosby, 1969:103–127.

4. Schepens CL. Retinal detachment and allied diseases. Philadelphia: WB Saunders, 1983:139–140.

5. Straatsma BR, Foos RY, et al. Degenerative diseases of the peripheral retina. In: Duane TD, Jaeger EA, eds. Clinical ophthalmology, vol. 3. Philadelphia: Harper & Row, 1980;26:20–24.

6. Foos RY. Zonular traction tufts of the peripheral retina in cadaver eyes. Arch Ophthalmol 1969;82:620–632.

7. Foos RY. Vitreous base, retinal tufts and retinal tears: pathological relationships. In: Pruitt RC, ed. Retina congress. New York: Appleton-Century-Crofts, 1974:259.

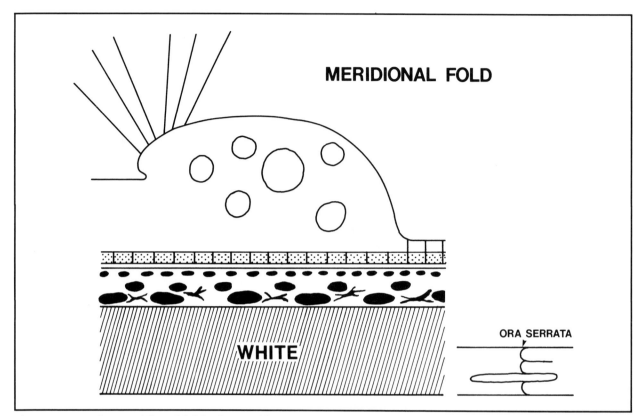

Figure 3.35 The meridional fold is located both in the retina and pars plana, shows cystoid degeneration, and has vitreous traction on the posterior end.

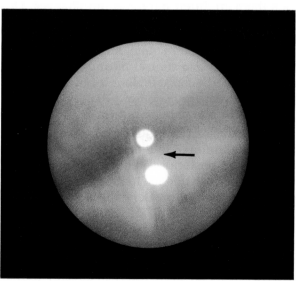

Figure 3.36 There is a small hole at the posterior end of a meridional fold (arrow), and signs of vitreous traction. The location is the superior nasal ora serrata, seen through the indirect condensing lens with scleral depression.

breaks. These breaks may be located anywhere along the edge of the fold and can lead to a rhegmatogenous retinal detachment. Breaks associated with meridional folds or the vitreous base are usually located in the upper half of the fundus, with the upper nasal quadrant being affected most frequently.[5] Meridional folds are not a common cause of retinal detachment, however.[2,6]

Periodic examinations should be performed with indirect ophthalmoscopy and a three-mirror contact lens to determine the existence of retinal breaks associated with meridional folds. Because of the anterior location of these lesions, cryopexy is the preferred treatment when a retinal break is present.

REFERENCES

1. Rutnin U, Schepens CL. Fundus appearance in normal eyes. II. The standard peripheral fundus and developmental variation. Am J Ophthalmol 1967;64:840–852.
2. Spencer LM, Foos RY, et al. Meridional folds, meridional complexes and associated abnormalities of the peripheral retina. Am J Ophthalmol 1970;70:697–718.
3. Schepens CL. Retinal detachment and allied diseases. Philadelphia: WB Saunders, 1983:139.
4. Straatsma BR, Foos RY, et al. Degenerative diseases of the peripheral retina. In: Duane TD, Jaeger EA, eds. Clinical ophthalmology, vol. 3. Philadelphia: Harper & Row, 1980;26:5–6.
5. Pischel DK. Retinal detachment: a manual, ed. 2. Am Acad Ophthalmol Otolaryngol, 1965;72.
6. Straatsma BR, Landers MB, et al. The ora serrata in the adult human eye. Arch Ophthalmol 1968;80:3–20.

Enclosed Ora Bay

Figure 3.37 Completely enclosed ora bay is isolated from the pars plana by two large ora teeth that unite anterior to the enclosed bay. Note the small retinal erosion at the posterior edge of the enclosed bay (arrow). View is through the indirect condensing lens with scleral depression.

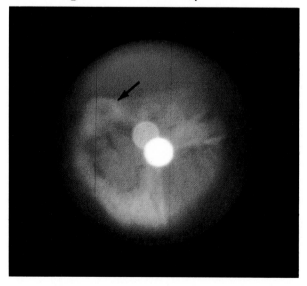

An enclosed ora bay, also known as a ring tooth or hole-in-a-tooth,[1] results from the enclosing of an island of pars plana by peripheral retina at the ora serrata.

CLINICAL DESCRIPTION

The ora bay can be partially or totally enclosed. A partially enclosed ora bay or open ring is produced when two adjacent teeth come close to each other but never unite (Figure 3.38A). A totally enclosed ora bay can be produced by two slender adjacent teeth uniting at their anterior apices—ring tooth—or if two adjacent teeth merge to form one large tooth "hole-in-the-tooth" (Figures 3.37 and 3.38B).

Enclosed ora bays are brownish depressions surrounded by normal-appearing retina, frequently displaying cystoid degeneration. Enclosed ora bays occur in about 3% to 4% of all eyes and 6% of all patients, and are bilateral in 8% of affected individuals.[2-4] A ring tooth is found in 2% of eyes.[5] In two studies, 73% of enclosed bays were associated with a meridional complex in the same clock position and sometimes a bay was part of a complex; also, 20% of enclosed bays had a meridional fold immediately anterior or posterior to them.[4,5] They are usually located near the horizontal meridian and occur equally between the nasal and temporal halves of the fundus.[4,5]

HISTOPATHOLOGY

An enclosed ora bay is composed of a thin layer of pars plana surrounded by sensory retina (Figure 3.38).

CLINICAL SIGNIFICANCE

An enclosed ora bay may be mistaken for a retinal hole; however, careful examination with indirect ophthalmoscopy or a three-mirror contact lens will reveal the brownish color of the pars plana island. A retinal erosion or full-thickness break may be found immediately posterior

Figure 3.38 Enclosed ora bay. Note that the enclosed bay is isolated from the pars plana by peripheral retina. (A) Partially enclosed bay. (B) Totally enclosed bay.

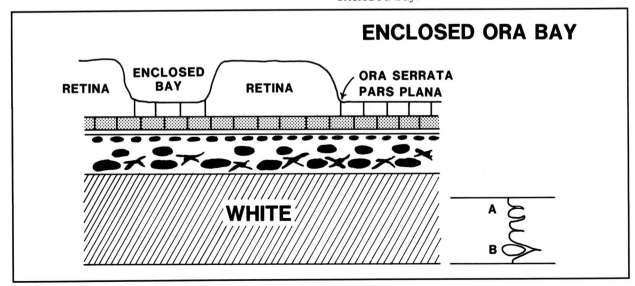

to an enclosed bay (Figure 3.37). Retinal breaks may occur in one out of six enclosed ora bays at the posterior edge. These were found in 16.7% of all eyes,[4] and all were associated with a posterior vitreous detachment.

REFERENCES

1. Schepens CL. Retinal detachment and allied diseases. Philadelphia: WB Saunders, 1983; 8:137–138.
2. Straatsma BR, Foos RY, et al. Degenerative diseases of the peripheral retina. In: Duane TD, Jaeger EA, eds. Clinical ophthalmology, vol. 3. Philadelphia: Harper & Row, 1980;26:7.
3. Rutnin U, Schepens CL. Fundus appearance in normal eyes. IV. Retinal breaks and other findings. Am J Ophthalmol 1967;64:1063–1078.
4. Spencer LM, Foos RY, et al. Enclosed ora bays of the ora serrata: relationship to retinal tears. Arch Ophthalmol 1970;83:421–425.
5. Spencer LM, Foos RY, et al. Meridional folds, meridional complexes, and associated abnormalities of the peripheral retina. Am J Ophthalmol 1970;70:697–714.

Pearls of the Ora Serrata

CLINICAL DESCRIPTION

Pearls of the ora serrata are bright glistening white spheroids on the dentate processes (Figure 3.39). They are usually single and are located between the base and the tip of the dentate process. In the early stage of development, they appear as dark brown, round bodies in an ora tooth due to the covering of the pigment epithelium. Later they become highly visible when the pigment epithelium over the pearl becomes thinned or absent.

Ora pearls occur in any quadrant of the fundus and approximately 20% of 700 consecutive studied autopsied eyes had a recognizable pearl. If both eyes were examined, there was a

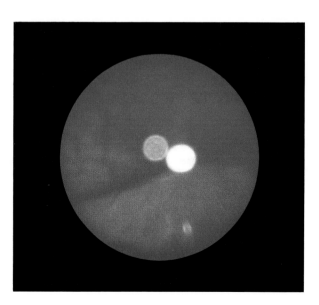

Figure 3.39 Small ora pearl can be seen on the ora serrata through the indirect condensing lens.

Chorioretinal Atrophy (Paving-Stone Degeneration)

Figure 3.41 Paving-stone degeneration in the inferior fundus. Note that the large and medium-sized choroidal vessels are seen more easily through the lesions and that there is pigment on the edges and in the center of the lesions.

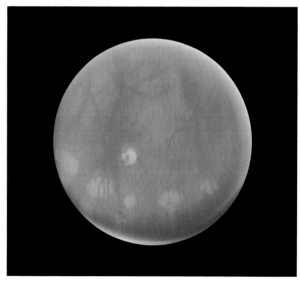

CLINICAL DESCRIPTION

Chorioretinal atrophy usually appears as round, depigmented areas in the retina in which a clear view of the medium- and large-sized vessels of the choroid are seen against the white background of the sclera. They usually vary from 0.1 to 1.5 mm, but occasionally are many disc diameters in size. Pigment can be found at the edges, on incomplete septa, or in the centers of these lesions.[1] Small lesions may coalesce into large areas with convex scalloped margins and incomplete septa. When the lesions are aligned in a row parallel to the ora serrata, the condition is known as paving-stone or cobblestone degeneration (Figures 2.3, 3.41, and 3.42).

Paving-stone degeneration is present in 22% of adults[2] and their prevalence increases markedly with age, from 10% in persons in their twenties to more than 30% of those greater than 70 years of age.[1,3] There seems to be a preference for the inferior region of the fundus and more than half of these lesions are located between the five and seven o'clock positions.[1] They are bilateral in 38% of autopsied eyes.[4] The majority are found just posterior to the ora serrata; rarely they occur as far posterior as the equator. They can, however, occasionally be seen in the posterior pole and pars plana. Chorioretinal degeneration and atrophy can affect the same areas of the peripheral retina. Chorioretinal atrophy is believed to be the result of the occlusion of a single lobule of choroidal circulation that produces a focal postischemic atrophy of the pigment epithelium and outer layers of the sensory retina.

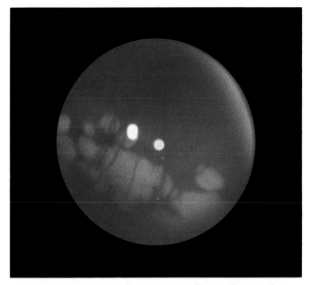

Figure 3.42 A much more confluent form of paving-stone degeneration in the inferior nasal fundus seen through the indirect condensing lens.

Figure 3.43 The chorioretinal atrophy shows a loss of the choriocapillaris and the outer four layers of the retina, resulting in loss of tissue and small depression of the retina. Loss of pigment epithelium and choriocapillaris allows a clear view of the choroid and sclera. There can be pigment epithelial hyperplasia at the edges of the lesion and pigment migration from the degenerated pigment epithelium into the sensory retina.

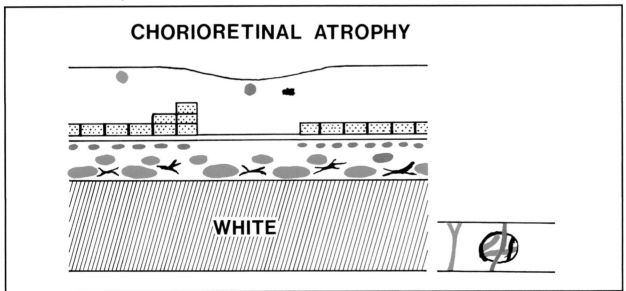

HISTOPATHOLOGY

The pathology appears to result from the closure of small areas of the choriocapillaris, which produces subsequent atrophy of the overlying pigment epithelium and outer layers of the sensory retina (Figure 3.43). There is loss of photoreceptors and the external limiting membrane. All of the above retinal layers are nourished by the choriocapillaris. The inner layers of the retina are essentially intact, since the retinal circulation supplies these layers. Thus there is a clear windowlike view of the choroid and sclera through the intact inner retinal layers. The inner surface of these lesions is slightly depressed as a result of tissue loss in the choroid and retina. The pigmented borders and septa are the result of the proliferation of pigment epithelial cells at the edges of the lesions. Other pigmented areas may be the result of pigment migration from the degenerated pigment epithelial cells that were within the boundaries of the chorioretinal atrophy. The remaining inner retinal layers become tightly adherent to the basal lamina (Bruch's membrane), which may show damage in its inner layers.

CLINICAL SIGNIFICANCE

Since the inner retinal layers are spared in the degenerative process, there are no breaks through which fluid can penetrate into the subretinal region to produce a retinal detachment. Therefore these lesions do not predispose to retinal detachment. If a retinal detachment involves an area of chorioretinal atrophy, however, the tight adherence to the basal lamina may produce a tear in the retina at the edge of the lesion. These breaks are often small and irregular in shape, and close examination may be necessary to detect them.

REFERENCES

1.   O'Malley PF, Allen RA, et al. Paving-stone degeneration of the retina. Arch Ophthalmol 1965;73:169–182.
2.   Straatsma BR, Foos RY, et al. Degenerative diseases of the peripheral retina. In: Duane TD, Jaeger EA, eds. Clinical ophthalmology, vol. 3. Philadelphia: Harper & Row, 1980;26:13–15.
3.   Rutnin U, Schepens CL, Fundus appearance in normal eyes. II. The standard peripheral fundus and developmental variations. Am J Ophthalmol 1967;64:840–852.
4.   Yanoff M, Fine BS, Ocular pathology: a text and atlas. Second edition. Philadelphia: Harper & Row, 1982:513.

White-With or
-Without-Pressure

CLINICAL DESCRIPTION

White-with-pressure is an optical phenomenon in which the fundus changes from its usually orange-red color to a translucent grayish white upon scleral depression (Figure 3.44). White-without-pressure has the same appearance without the physical application of scleral indention (Figures 2.3 and 3.45). This condition can occur in a small isolated area or be seen as a circumferential band that travels the entire perimeter of the retina. The circumferential band can have smooth or scalloped margins. The area of white-with or -without-pressure can be migratory in nature and therefore its shape can be different on subsequent examinations.[1] The posterior margin of this condition tends to be very sharp and the anterior margin gently fades into the peripheral retina. It is not unusual to see just posterior to an area of white-without-pressure a small zone where the retina appears to

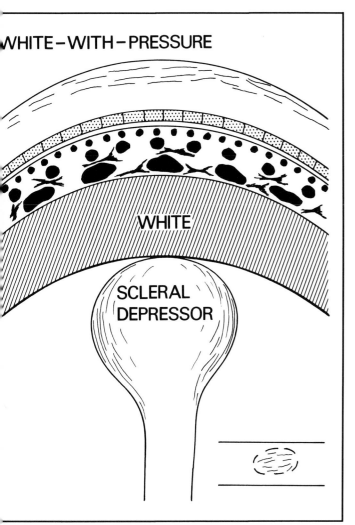

WHITE–WITH–PRESSURE

WHITE

SCLERAL DEPRESSOR

Figure 3.44 White-with-pressure is produced by pushing an area of mild retinal degeneration into the vitreous cavity with a scleral depressor.

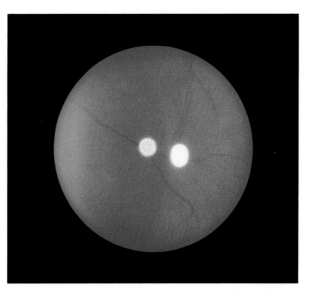

Figure 3.45 An area of white-without-pressure can be seen as a whitish patch peripheral in the fundus with a sharp demarcation line. The area is the nasal fundus seen through the indirect condensing lens.

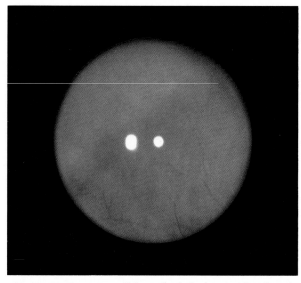

Figure 3.46 A small band of darker red retina is seen immediately posterior to an area of white-without-pressure. The area is the nasal fundus seen through the indirect condensing lens.

Figure 3.47 An island of normal-appearing retina is surrounded by white-without-pressure.

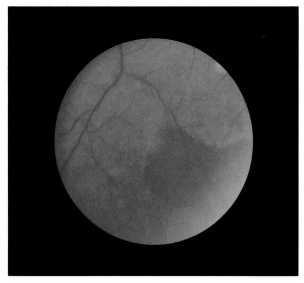

be darker red (Figure 3.46). The etiology of this dark zone is presumed to be the same as that of white-without-pressure. This condition is generally found from the ora serrata to approximately three disc diameters posteriorly; however, it can occur as far posterior as the equator and rarely, as far as the temporal arcades.

White-with or -without-pressure is presumed to be an optical phenomenon associated with the vitreoretinal interface. It is believed that continued mild vitreal traction is responsible for changes in the transparency of this interface. These areas of vitreoretinal adhesion may be portions of the vitreous base that are located further posterior than usual. There have been reports in the literature of mild retinal degeneration with loss of retinal transparency found in an area of white-without-pressure.[2] These degenerative findings may be the result of this condition occurring over prolonged periods of time. Loss of transparency may be fairly mild initially and may only be detected upon scleral depression.

Vitreous changes that may be associated with this condition are a posterior vitreous detachment with collapse or extensive liquefaction of the middle and posterior vitreous body (see Chapter 4). In either case, tractional forces are produced on the peripheral retina with subsequent degeneration.

White-with or -without-pressure is found to some extent in over 30% of normal eyes, with a strong tendency toward bilaterality. Individuals under 20 years of age have only a 5% occurrence, while those over 70 years of age have approximately a 66% frequency.[3] It most frequently occurs in myopes and the elderly, which is probably related to the increased vitreous degeneration in these individuals. It generally occurs in the superior or temporal regions of the fundus, and it is not uncommon to see this condition on the posterior edge of lattice degeneration and on the edge of a posterior staphyloma.

Figure 3.48 Operculated retinal tear with a large drusen next to it (arrowhead). The operculum is still attached to the detached vitreous (arrow). View is through the indirect condensing lens of the nasal fundus.

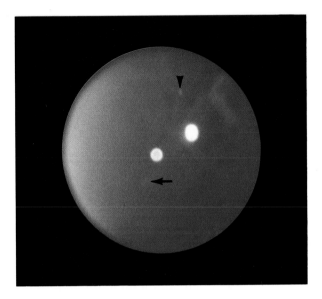

White-with or -without-pressure can have an island of normal-appearing retina within its borders (Figure 3.47). This is sometimes mistaken for a retinal tear surrounded by a retinal detachment. It can be differentiated from a true retinal break and detachment with the use of scleral depression or a three-mirror contact lens examination. With either procedure, the observer notices the absence of retinal elevation or torn edges of the suspected tear.

When a retinal break is not very evident on ophthalmoscopy, its appearance can be enhanced with scleral depression (Figures 3.48 and 3.49). Retinal breaks tend to be located in areas of retinal degeneration and if the degeneration is mild, white-with-pressure may help locate such areas during scleral depression. Scleral depression is recommended in areas of the fundus where vitreous floaters are found, in order to see if they originated from a barely visible retinal break. A pseudo-white-with-pressure can be seen in infants or in persons with darkly pigmented fundi, and has a watered-silk appearance.

Figure 3.49 Scleral depression of the retinal break demonstrates the white-with-pressure phenomenon, which is seen as a white halo around the hole. View is through the indirect condensing lens.

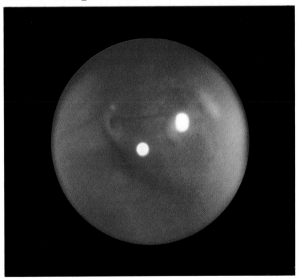

HISTOPATHOLOGY

White-with or -without-pressure gives a thinned and atrophic appearance to the retina (Figure 3.50). In one histologic study, the inner limiting membrane was disrupted or absent, the neural elements were disorganized, and the pigment epithelium was disrupted with evidence of pigment proliferation and migration.[2] There was also a layer of fluid between the pigment

Peripheral Cystoid
Degeneration

CLINICAL DESCRIPTION

Peripheral cystoid degeneration appears as translucent red dots within an area with grayish white margins. It is composed of a band of intraretinal cystoid cavities that are usually found about one-half a disc diameter from the ora serrata (see Figures 2.3 and 2.10), but they can extend as far posteriorly as the equator. The involved retina has up to three times its normal thickness. The surface has small white depressions that are the ends of the pillars between the intervening round domes, which are the inner walls of the cystoid spaces. The cystoid spaces appear reddish due to the increased visibility of the choroidal reflex during ophthalmoscopy.[1] Dentate processes are commonly involved in cystoid degeneration.

Peripheral cystoid degeneration occurs more frequently in the temporal half of the retina than the nasal half, and more frequently on the superior than the inferior half.[2] It appears to begin next to the ora serrata and slowly spreads posteriorly. There can be changes in the vitreous above cystoid degeneration consisting of vitreous strands and grayish opacities that sometimes resemble snowflakes.

There are two types of peripheral cystoid degeneration, typical and reticular. Typical cystoid degeneration appears as dark reddish dots that may coalesce to form interlacing tunnels (see Figure 3.53). This form occurs bilaterally and is seen in all patients over 8 years old and increases with age.[3] It has been found in infants as young as 1 year of age. Typical cystoid is most frequently found in the superior and temporal quadrants.

Reticular cystoid degeneration appears as a finely stippled surface with a linear reticular pattern that corresponds to sclerotic retinal vessels. The involved areas may be single or multiple and they are irregular in shape with sharp angular margins. The posterior limit of these patches is often demarcated by retinal blood vessels. Reticular cystoid degeneration is located posterior to and continuous with typical cystoid degeneration.

Reticular cystoid degeneration is found in 18% of the adult population and is bilateral in 41% of the cases.[4] It is most frequently seen in the inferior temporal quadrant. This condition occurs in persons in every decade of life and does not seem to be related to the aging process of the peripheral retina. An interesting theory with respect to the possible formation of peripheral cystoid degeneration is that it is caused by the traction and movement of the ora serrata during accommodation.[5]

HISTOPATHOLOGY

Typical cystoid degeneration begins as cystoid spaces in the outer plexiform and adjacent

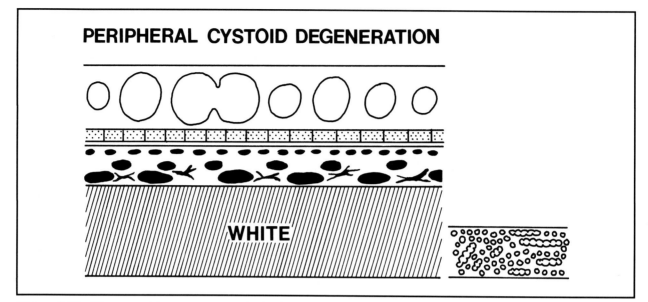

Figure 3.51   The cystoid process starts in the inner retinal layers and enlarges circumferentially. The pillars may break between the cystoid spaces.

nuclear layers of the retina (Figures 3.51 and 3.52).[6] With time, these cavities can extend from the inner to the outer limiting membrane. Cystoid cavities are separated by pillars composed of compressed Müller cells and photoreceptor axons. The cavities contain hyaluronic acid, which may represent degenerative neural tissue. The pillars may break, thus producing larger cystoid cavities, and a massive rupturing of these pillars may be the mechanism by which a retinoschisis is formed. Peripheral cystoid degeneration always occurs anterior to retinoschises. The pigment epithelium under cystoid degeneration does not show signs of involvement.[7]

Reticular cystoid degeneration begins as small cystoid spaces in the nerve fiber layer of the retina. With time, these cavities can extend from the inner limiting membrane to the outer plexiform layer. These smaller cystoid spaces in the inner layers of the retina are responsible for the finely stippled surface. These cavities are also filled with hyaluronic acid.[8]

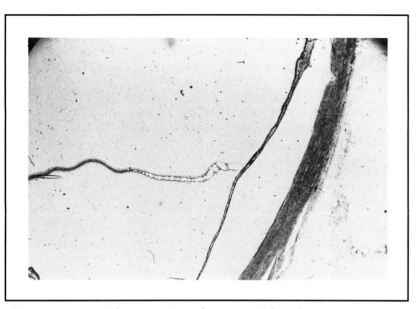

Figure 3.52 Histology section shows peripheral cystoid degeneration in an artifactually separated retina. Note that the peripheral cystoid spaces are larger and many of the interseptal pillars have broken, which may be the mechanism in the formation of a retinoschisis. The remnants of the pillars can be seen on the inner and outer walls, and those on the inner wall are possibly responsible for the phenomenon known as snowflakes on retinoschisis. Finally, note how thin the inner and outer walls become as the degeneration progresses.

CLINICAL SIGNIFICANCE

Retinal holes can develop in peripheral cystoid degeneration and they are usually the result of a rupture of the inner wall of a cystoid cavity (Figures 3.53 and 3.54). The inner wall of the cavity is thinner than the outer wall, making it more susceptible to rupturing. The outer wall usually remains intact, and thus liquefied vitreous is only able to fill the cavity itself. Therefore retinal holes in cystoid degeneration generally do not require treatment since they

Figure 3.53 A red retinal hole with a small surrounding retinal detachment in an area of peripheral cystoid degeneration. The lesion above the hole is a cryopexy scar from a previously treated retinal hole.

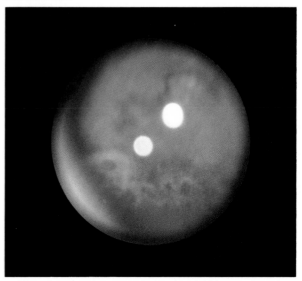

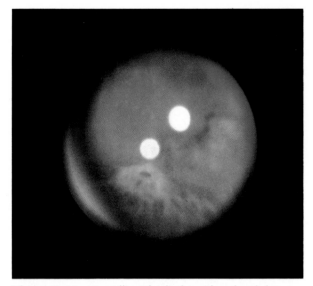

Figure 3.54 By rolling the hole with scleral depression, the posterior edge of the hole can be detected. The area is the inferior retina viewed through the indirect condensing lens.

usually do not produce a retinal detachment. If there is a rupture in both the outer and inner walls of the cystoid cavity, a retinal detachment can occur. There have been a few reports in the literature of a retinal detachment being caused by a hole in cystoid degeneration.

The other clinically significant aspect of peripheral cystoid degeneration is its possible implication in the formation of a retinoschisis (see page 87).

REFERENCES

1. Hines JL, Jones WL. Peripheral microcystoid retinal degeneration and retinoschisis. J Am Optom Assoc 1982;53:541–545.
2. Straatsma BR, Foos RY. Typical and reticular degenerative retinoschisis. Am J Opthalmol 1973;75:551–575.
3. O'Malley PF, Allen RA. Peripheral cystoid degeneration of the retina: incidence and distribution in 1,000 autopsy eyes. Arch Ophthalmol 1967;77:769–776.
4. Straatsma BR, Foos RY, et al. Degenerative diseases of the peripheral retina. In: Duane TD, Jaeger EA, eds. Clinical ophthalmology, vol. 3. Philadelphia: Harper & Row, 1980;26:8–10.
5. Teng CC, Katzen HM. An anatomic study of the periphery of the retina. II. Peripheral cystoid degeneration of the retina: formation of cysts and holes. Am J Ophthalmol 1953;36:29–39.
6. Gottinger W. Senile retinoschisis. Stuttgart: Georg Thieme, 1978.
7. Foos RY. Senile retinoschisis: relationship to cystoid degeneration. Trans Am Acad Ophthalmol Otolaryngol 1970;74:33–51.
8. Yanoff M, Fine BS. Ocular pathology: a text and atlas, ed. 2. Philadelphia: Harper & Row, 1982:504–505.

Retinoschisis

Retinoschisis results from the splitting of the sensory retina into two layers. It may be congenital or acquired and although the physical appearance is essentially the same, the pathogenesis of the two forms is different.

CLINICAL DESCRIPTION

Acquired retinoschisis, also known as senile or adult retinoschisis, is a separation of the sensory retina at the outer plexiform and inner nuclear layers. It is most often found in the temporal half of the fundus, especially the inferior temporal region (about 70%) and about 25% in the superior temporal quadrant. Acquired retinoschisis is seen in about 4% of persons.[1] It is commonly found in those 40 years of age or older and it is rare under the age of 20 years.[2-4] It seems to occur more frequently in females.[5] Advanced retinoschisis is found in approxi-

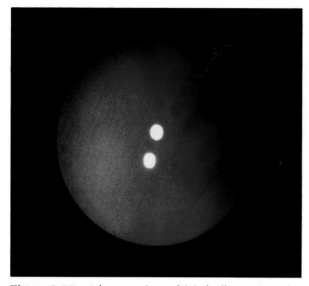

Figure 3.55 A large retinoschisis balloons into the vitreous cavity from the temporal fundus seen through the indirect condensing lens. Note that the schisis has a smooth, taut surface and that it is fairly transparent.

Figure 3.56 B-scan ultrasonogram of retinoschisis seen in Figure 3.55. Note the small sonic echo sent back by the thin inner layer of the schisis. White striated area on the left is feedback noise from the eyelid to the transducer.

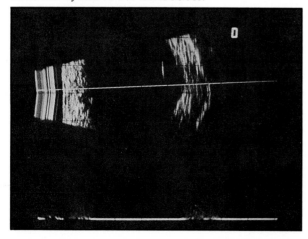

mately 7% of persons over 40 years of age.[6] This condition tends to be bilateral (82.1%)[4] and symmetric. It usually is not considered to be inherited, but some authors believe that advanced retinoschisis may be transmitted by an autosomal recessive or incomplete dominant trait.[7]

Retinoschisis is typically seen as an elevated bullous lesion in the peripheral fundus (Figures 2.10 and 3.55). It has a smooth, taut surface that does not undulate on eye movements, as commonly occurs with retinal detachments. The inner layer of the schisis is very thin, as shown by ultrasonography (Figure 3.56) and it can be essentially transparent to fairly translucent. Many times the detection of a schisis depends on the observation of blood vessels traversing upward into the vitreous cavity in the inner layer of the lesion (Figure 3.57).[8] Sometimes retinal vessels can be found in the outer layer of the schisis and they may be stretched between the two layers. Such a vessel may rupture and fill the schisis cavity with a layered hemorrhage.[6] Frequently, occluded, white, sclerotic vessels are present in the inner layer, which helps in the differential diagnosis between a schisis and a detachment (Figure 3.58).

Tiny snowflakes can be present on the surface of 70% of lesions.[9] They are either the result of condensation of the vitreous onto the inner layer or remnants of glial pillars attached to the inner wall (Figure 3.59). Snowflakes are usually found on the posterior portion of the schisis, on or just internal to the inner layer. Sometimes a schisis is detected only after the discovery of snowflakes that seem to be floating in the vitreous over the peripheral retina.

Both the inner and outer layers of a schisis may have a honeycomb or beaten-metal appearance, especially when viewed with a three-mirror contact lens or during indirect ophthalmoscopy with scleral depression. The outer layer covers the choroid with a faint haze and breaks in the layer appear as pinkish round areas. The appearance of a group of these outer layer breaks is sometimes called "frog's eggs."[6] Rarely, pigmented or white demarcation lines occur along the posterior margin of a schisis (Figure 2.10); however, such lines are much more frequently associated with retinal detachments (A patient with bilateral superior temporal schisis with multiple pigmented demarcation lines in the inner layers was seen by WLJ) (see Demarcation Lines, page 188). We have seen incidences of a small retinal hemorrhage at the posterior margin of a retinoschisis on two occasions (Figure 3.58) and a case of an extensive vitreous hemorrhage secondary to an acquired retinoschisis. This is believed to be a result of vitreous traction or the acute angulation of retinal vessels as they travel onto the schisis.

Peripheral cystoid degeneration is always found between the anterior edge of the schisis and the ora serrata. The pathogenesis of a schisis seems to be associated closely with cystoid degeneration. The pillars between the cystoid spaces break with progressive degeneration (Figure 3.52) and a massive coalescence of these spaces is what most authorities believe causes a retinoschisis. It can be very difficult to determine clinically where peripheral cystoid degeneration stops and retinoschisis begins.

Vitreous degeneration is almost always found in association with acquired retinoschisis. It consists of liquefaction of the vitreous gel and posterior vitreous detachment (PVD), which occurs in 60% of cases.[2] The vitreous gel next to the schisis often displays prominent, taut fibers, some of which are not attached to the inner layer of the schisis and appear large and

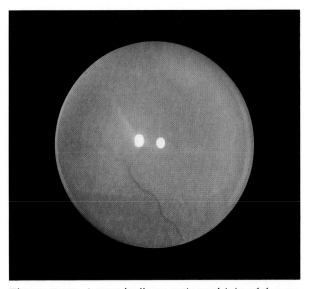

Figure 3.57 Large bullous retinoschisis of the superior fundus seen through the indirect condensing lens. Note that the retinal blood vessels travel upward in the inner layer of the posterior region of the schisis.

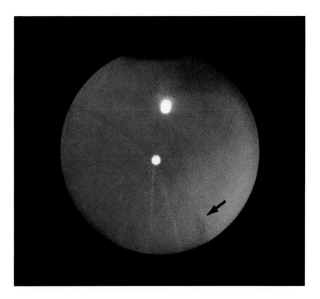

Figure 3.58 A bullous retinoschisis in the superior temporal fundus seen through the indirect condensing lens. Note the white sclerotic retinal vessel traveling upward onto the schisis and the small retinal hemorrhage at the posterior margin of the schisis (arrow).

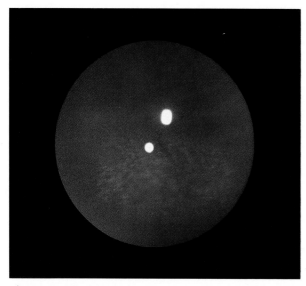

Figure 3.59 Very transparent retinoschisis with numerous snowflakes on the inner surface in the superior temporal fundus seen through the indirect condensing lens.

curled. This is one explanation for the clinical finding of snowflakes. The liquefied vitreous gel becomes a potential source of fluid that enters breaks in the retinoschisis and possibly produces a retinal detachment. Breaks in the inner layer of the schisis may be associated with a PVD, and a retinal detachment produced by breaks in the inner and outer layers is almost always associated with a PVD in the region of the inner layer break.[10]

Most patients with an acquired retinoschisis are asymptomatic until the lesion is in an advanced stage. Possible symptoms are flashes and floaters, peripheral field defects, and decreased acuity. The flashes and floaters are the result of vitreous traction. The visual field defects are absolute and progress with advancement of the schisis. This compares to a relative visual field defect that is found in a retinal detachment. Often, however, there is no visual field defect detected unless the schisis is posterior to the equator.[1,11] Visual acuity may be reduced if a peripheral schisis invades the macula (a rare occurrence), if an associated retinal detachment involves the macula, or if there is cystoid macular degeneration associated with a temporal retinoschisis. Also, there are reported incidences of a perifoveal retinoschisis associated with peripheral schisis. In such a case, the patient may have 20/20 foveal vision with a perifoveal scotoma.[6]

Progression of a retinoschisis is very slow and is probably the result of the slow degenerative process of peripheral cystoid degeneration together with the viscous nature of the fluid within the cavity. It seems to grow in a circular and posterior direction, and becomes elevated. Most retinoschises become stationary or progress very slowly. One study of 245 eyes found that only 13.5% had documented growth when observed over a time period of 1 month to 15 years.[12] Sometimes a schisis will advance from the periphery to the posterior pole and then remain stationary for years. Progression results from either continued vitreous traction or from a secretory mechanism that produces more fluid in the cavity of the schisis. There have been cases reported in which once vitreous traction was relieved from the inner layer of a schisis, progression ceased.[10] Therefore vitreous traction may be the most important factor in progression.

A traction retinoschisis occurs as the result of marked vitreous traction that physically pulls the sensory retina into two layers. Its clinical appearance is the same as that of the acquired form, except that there are large vitreous bands attached to the inner layer of the schisis; these advance very slowly or remain stationary. Traction retinoschises occur in eyes that are often afflicted with severe uveitis, proliferative diabetic retinopathy, recurrent vitreous hemorrhages, vitreous scarring secondary to trauma, and retrolental fibroplasia.

Congenital retinoschisis (also known as juvenile retinoschisis, juvenile ideopathic retinoschisis, and juvenile sex-link retinoschisis) is transmitted as a sex-linked recessive trait and therefore is found exclusively in males. There have been rare cases where it has occurred in females as an autosomal recessive disease.[12,13] The condition is usually first discovered in young adults and children but it may be present at birth.[5] Patients generally complain of seeing floaters, decreased vision, nystagmus, and strabismus. In the absence of vitreous hemorrhage, visual acuity may be 20/40 or better, but often drops below 20/70, and tends to stabilize at 20/200 or worse.[6] In over half of patients, visual acuity is worse than 20/70. Bilaterality is the rule; however, the degree of involvement in the contralateral eye can vary.

Congenital retinoschisis is usually found in the inferior temporal quadrant and it may extend over two quadrants. Splitting of the sensory retina occurs in the nerve fiber layer and the ballooning schisis tends to be very transparent. The congenital form does not extend to the ora serrata and is not associated with extensive cystoid degeneration of the retina. White or pigmented demarcation lines are seen more frequently in congenital retinoschisis than in the acquired form. It is not uncommon for a vitreous hemorrhage to occur, probably as the result of vitreous traction on retinal vessels. The retinal vessels that traverse across the inner layer breaks may be at greater risk for hemorrhaging. The vitreous hemorrhage can set up a vicious cycle resulting in vitreous scarring and a further increase in vitreous traction. Vitreous hemorrhage is frequent in young patients but is rarely seen in persons over 20 years of age.[6]

Most cases of congenital retinoschisis are not discovered until patients reach 5 years of age, most likely due to the fact that the upper visual field is usually affected. Visual loss in the upper visual field is generally not appreciated by children nor does it greatly affect their visual performance. Progression of the disease is rapid in the first five years of life, after which it advances more slowly and usually becomes stationary by age 20 years.[6]

The pathogenesis of congenital retinoschisis appears to be inadequate growth of the vitreous gel that is unable to keep up with the circumferential growth of the retina, choroid, and sclera. Therefore tractional forces are applied to the young retina that causes a split in the nerve fiber layer.

The macula may be involved and appears as a starshaped area of cystic degeneration. Visual acuity is usually mildly to moderately affected. Despite cystic changes in the macula, fluorescein angiography rarely demonstrates macular edema in sex-linked retinoschisis, nor does it demonstrate angiographic anomalies in the senile variety. Macular involvement is either the direct result of peripheral schisis that is involving or has involved the macula, or it may occur independent of peripheral schisis formation. No treatment seems to help this macular condition.[6]

HISTOPATHOLOGY

Acquired forms of retinoschisis appear as large cystic cavities in the sensory retina that result from the splitting of the sensory retina at the outer plexiform and inner nuclear layers (Figure 3.60). The inner layer is usually extremely thin and contains patent and hyalinized blood vessels, glial cells, remnants of the inner nuclear and nerve fiber layers, and the internal limiting membrane. Remnants of the glial pillars may be found on the inner surface of the inner layer. The outer layer of the schisis is irregular

Figure 3.60   Note the intraretinal cavity that is filled with a viscous fluid and the extreme thinning of the inner and outer layers of the schisis. An inner layer hole appears clear and an outer layer hole looks red in the schisis.

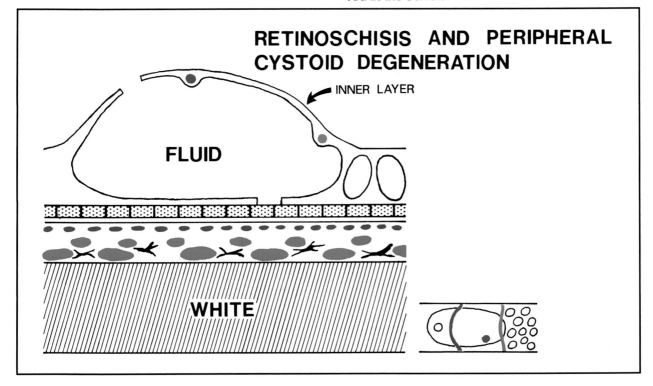

later they seem to be concentrated at the borders of the lesions.[12] They give the retinal surface of the lesion a granular appearance. It is not uncommon to find white-with or -without-pressure along the borders of the lesion (especially the posterior border), which is indicative of vitreous traction. Another condition that sometimes occurs concomitantly is chorioretinal atrophy.

The vitreous over areas of lattice degeneration shows liquefaction of the vitreous gel that forms a lacuna (Figure 3.68). The lacuna is lined by a condensation membrane of vitreous that is attached at the edges of the lattice lesion. Posterior vitreous detachment is not uncommon

Figure 3.68 Lattice degeneration with sclerosed white vessels (center vessel is totally occluded), pigment migration into the sensory retina, a red atrophic hole, chorioretinal atrophy, a vitreous lacuna, and vitreous traction on the edges of the lesion. Note that the retina is degenerated to about one-third its normal thickness.

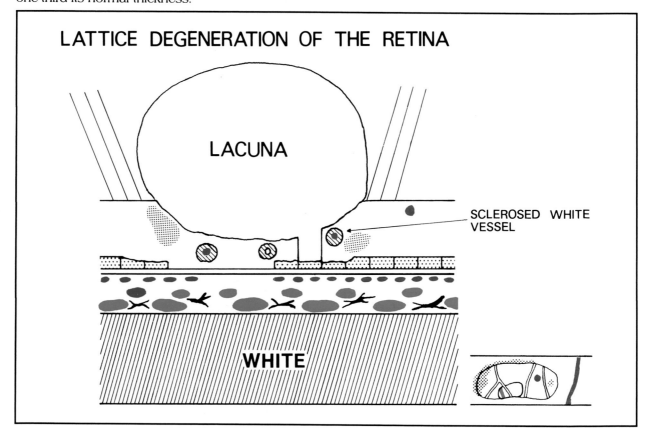

and it generally does not involve the area of lattice degeneration due to strong vitreoretinal adhesions. An early lattice lesion may have a small isolated lacuna over it, but an advanced lesion tends to have a large lacuna with communications to other lacunae within the vitreous body. This can make available a large quantity of liquefied vitreous to enter a retinal break and cause retinal detachment.

Lattice degeneration is a slowly progressive disease that results in gradual retinal thinning and loss of transparency. With time, there may appear within the lesion punched-out areas, retinal cysts and breaks, and occasionally, a small retinal hemorrhage.

Fluorescein angiography displays delayed filling of the retinal vessels in the lattice lesion but no leakage of dye outside the vessels.[2] Due to defects in the pigment epithelium, areas of hyperfluorescence—window defects—are seen in the lesion.

The pathogenesis of lattice degeneration may be localized retinal ischemia that produces retinal and vitreal degeneration, or the condition may primarily be the result of vitreous degeneration causing localized areas of vitreoretinal traction with secondary loss of inner retinal tissue. Another proposed theory is that of genetic predisposition and developmental factors.[8]

HISTOPATHOLOGY

Lattice degeneration shows variable retinal thinning, with the greatest amount generally in the center (Figure 3.68). The retinal surface is irregular and has amorphous gray-white particles.[11] There is loss of the inner retinal layers down to the outer nuclear and outer limiting membranes that are often replaced in part by glial elements. There is often a conspicuous loss of photoreceptors within the lesion.[13] Advanced

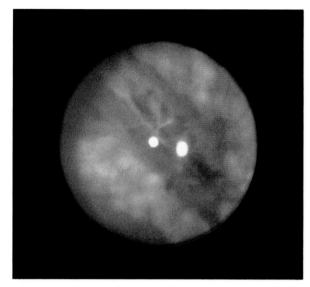

Figure 3.72 Fresh argon laser photocoagulation spots are bright white areas around the perivascular lattice degeneration shown in Figures 3.65 and 3.70. The view is through the indirect condensing lens.

Management of lattice degeneration with breaks is to record the location and pertinent characteristics of the lesion and follow the patient on a yearly basis. Patients with symptoms of floaters and photopsia must be examined at six-month intervals. It is important to perform the examination with binocular indirect ophthalmoscopy and scleral depression. Patients with asymptomatic small retinal holes need not be treated unless there are coexisting circumstances that enhance the possibility of a retinal detachment, such as aphakia, high myopia, vitreous scarring, etc. Treatment is generally required if retinal tears exist in or near the lattice lesion.

The treatment of lattice degeneration with significant breaks and without a retinal detachment is photocoagulation (Figure 3.72) and cryopexy. The development of a retinal detachment requires the additional procedure of scleral buckling with or without an encircling band.

REFERENCES

1. Boniuk M, Butler FC. An autopsy study of lattice degeneration, retinal breaks and retinal pits. In: McPherson A, ed. New and controversial aspects of retinal detachment. New York: Harper & Row, 1968:59–75.
2. Straatsma BR, Zeegen PD, et al. Lattice degeneration of the retina. Trans Am Acad Ophthalmol Otolaryngol 1974;78:87–113.
3. Everett WG. Bilateral retinal detachment and degeneration. Trans Am Ophthalmol Soc 1966;64:543–585.
4. Halpern JI. Routine screening of the retinal periphery. Am J Ophthalmol 1966;62:99–102.
5. Beyer NE. Clinical study of lattice degeneration of the retina. Trans Am Acad Ophthalmol Otolaryngol 1965;69:1064–1081.
6. Beyer NE. Changes in and prognosis of lattice degeneration of the retina. Trans Am Acad Ophthalmol Otolaryngol 1974;78:114–125.
7. Straatsma BR, Zeegen PD, et al. Lattice degen-

eration of the retina. Trans Am Acad Ophthalmol Otolaryngol 1974;77:619–649.

8. Straatsma BR, Allen RA. Lattice degeneration of the retina. Trans Am Acad Ophthalmol Otolaryngol 1962;66:600–613.

9. Schepens CL. Retinal detachment and allied diseases. Philadelphia: WB Saunders, 1983; 8:167–169.

10. Gartner J. Erbbedingte aquatoriale degenerationen nictmyoper. Solitarformen und oraparallele bander. Klin Monatsbl Augenheilkd 1960; 136:523–539.

11. Tolentino FI, Schepens CL, et al. Vitreoretinal disorders; diagnosis and management. Philadelphia: WB Saunders, 1976;16:340–349.

12. Beyer NE. Lattice degeneration of the retina. Surv Ophthalmol 1979;23:213–248.

13. Yanoff M, Fine BS. Ocular pathology: a text and atlas, ed. 2. Philadelphia: Harper & Row, 1982;11:567–569.

14. Foss RY. retinal holes. Am J Ophthalmol 1978; 86:354–358.

15. Tillery WV, Lucier AC. Round atrophic holes in lattice degeneration—an important cause of aphakic retinal detachment. Trans Am Acad Ophthalmol Otolaryngol 1976;81:509–518.

16. Morse PH, Sheie HG. Prophylactic cryoretinopexy of retinal breaks. Arch Ophthalmol 1974; 92:204–207.

17. Straatsma BR, Zeegen PD, et al. Lattice degeneration of the retina. Am J Ophthalmol 1974; 77:619–649.

18. Dumas J, Schepens CL. Chorioretinal lesions predisposing to retinal breaks. Am J Ophthalmol 1966;61:620–630.

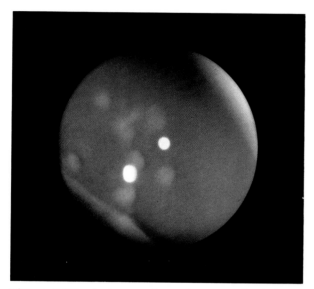

Figure 3.80 A group of exudates on the inferior temporal retina just posterior to the ora serrata in a patient with pars planitis. View is through an indirect condensing lens.

Figure 3.81 Slit-lamp view of anterior vitreous shows numerous white blood cells and a few vitreous strands in a patient with pars planitis.

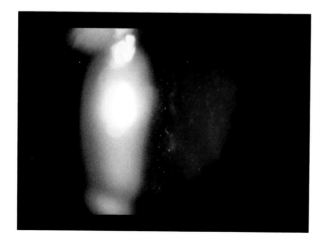

balls—on the peripheral retina, ora serrata, or pars plana (Figure 3.80). These exudates are most frequently found in the inferior region of the fundus, presumably due to gravitational forces. Inflammation results in the presence of white cells in the anterior vitreous (Figure 3.81). Sometimes a snowball opacity can be seen floating in the vitreous and may cause the patient to see a dark floater in the field of vision (Figure 3.82). There is often a peripheral vasculitis, usually affecting the veins, that is seen as attenuated and sheathed retinal vessels. Progression of the disease can lead to a continued obliteration of the vessels toward the posterior pole together with the development of optic atrophy and severe loss of vision.

Further progression leads to a coalescence of these exudates into a plaque—"snowbank"—that covers the ora serrata and hides all underlying detail (Figure 3.83). When the inflammation is active, the snowbank has a soft and slightly raised appearance but in quiescent stages it has a thin and membranous appearance. In advanced stages, there can be neovascularization of this membrane.[5]

Other ocular findings include yellowish, gelatinous exudates on the trabeculum of the filtration angle in 20% of cases.[6] Exudates can also occur on the anterior surface of the iris and peripheral anterior synechiae are often noted. In severe cases, a cyclitic membrane may develop behind the iris. Cataracts, usually posterior subcapsular occur frequently, the result of chronic inflammation and corticosteroid treatment.

Pars planitis is a chronic smoldering disease with remissions and exacerbations, which may last for 20 to 30 years. Some areas of the peripheral fundus may demonstrate active inflammatory deposits while others appear quiescent. The five-year projected visual prognosis is excellent for 80% of patients without treatment. Most of the remaining 20% do well on alternate-day oral prednisone or periocular steroid injections.[4]

The etiology of pars planitis is unknown, but an autoimmune mechanism is suggested at this time. One experimental study proposed that patients might be allergic to their own retina[7] and another suggested an immune reaction to vitreous cells.[8] There have been reports in the literature describing a relationship between pars planitis and multiple sclerosis.[9,10] The hyposensitivity of these patients to skin tests suggests a decrease in cell-mediated immunity that is also seen in lepromatous leprosy and sarcoid.[11] There have been reports of familial occurrence of pars planitis.[12]

HISTOPATHOLOGY

Pars planitis is a chronic granulomatous inflammation of the anterior retina and the pars plana ciliaris (Figure 3.84). There is vasculitis of the retinal vessels and often a periphlebitis is seen. The snowbank is composed of a loose fibrovascular layer containing occasional fibrocyte-like cells adjacent to hyperplastic nonpigmented epithelium of the pars plana.[13]

CLINICAL SIGNIFICANCE

Vitreous degeneration with subsequent shrinkage can produce tractional forces that may result in retinal folds and breaks. These retinal breaks can be operculated, linear, or horseshoe tears or retinal dialyses. Proliferation of the membrane at the vitreous base in a posterior direction may result in a sealing off of breaks, thus preventing a retinal detachment.[14]

Rhegmatogenous retinal detachments are noted in about 50% of cases. Exudative retinal detachments and choroidal effusions can also occur in these eyes and it is not unusual to dis-

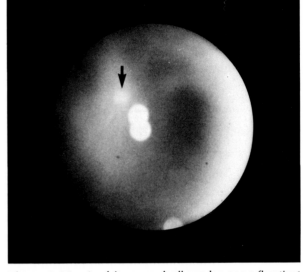

Figure 3.82 A white snowball can be seen floating in the vitreous of a patient with pars planitis (arrow). View is through an indirect condensing lens.

Figure 3.83 A bright white snowbank on the inferior ora serrata in a patient with pars planitis. View is through the indirect condensing lens with scleral depression.

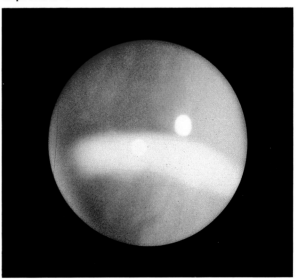

Posterior Vitreous Detachment

Figure 4.1 Posterior vitreous detachment with total collapse into the anterior vitreous cavity, seen during biomicroscopy. Note the sharp delineation of the posterior vitreous face against the optically dark liquefied vitreous.

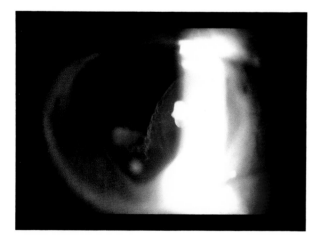

A posterior vitreous detachment (PVD) occurs when the vitreous cortex separates from the posterior retina and optic disc. If it extends to the ora serrata, it is known as a complete PVD (Figure 4.1); if it involves only a regional area it is known as an incomplete PVD. In adult eyes of all ages, occurrence is 2% for incomplete PVD and 12% for complete PVD. The frequency over age 65 years increases to 3% for incomplete and 31% for complete PVD. The PVD is symmetric in about 90% of the patients. In aphakic eyes at autopsy, incomplete PVD was seen in 6% and complete PVD in 66%.[1]

CLINICAL DESCRIPTION

The symptoms of a PVD are floaters, photopsia, blurred vision, and rarely, metamorphopsia. The posterior vitreous cortex is most adherent at the optic disc and macula and there is a gliotic ring at its attachment to the disc. It is common to see this avulsed gliotic ring floating in the vitreous after a PVD and it typically has an annular shape (Figure 4.2). It may be twisted into a figure-eight or other geometric form, however, or it may have a semicircular or linear shape when it is broken. Sometimes the glial tissue is not torn free in a PVD and no glial annulus is found. Rarely, a small gliotic annulus from the macula can be seen floating in the vitreous temporal to the larger annulus that originated from the optic disc. Floaters of many shapes and sizes are seen by the patient after a PVD, usually as the result of vitreous condensation and collapse, which produce discrete opacities that move about freely in liquefied vitreous. Floaters in the retrovitreous space may disappear from view due to gravitational migration into the inferior fundus, however, those in the detached vitreous face or in the cortex may persist for years.

Another cause of floaters is a vitreous hemorrhage that results from the rupture of a retinal vessel during a PVD. Tractional forces are to blame as the vitreous pulls away from the retina. These floaters are usually of sudden onset and are seen as many black specks against a bright background. Vitreous hemorrhages from a PVD are generally small and self-limiting. They are best seen during binocular indirect ophthalmoscopy as a faint plume of reddish smoke billowing into the vitreous. Vitreous hemorrhage occurs in 7.5% of all eyes with PVD and in 5% of patients with a symptomatic PVD without a retinal break.[2]

Photopsia (flashing lights) is the most frequent symptom and results from mechanical stimulation of the retina by the traction produced by the detaching vitreous. It is seen by patients 25% to 50% of the time.[3,4] Photopsia occurs during the active process of the PVD and only persists if areas of vitreoretinal attachment remain. The photopsia from these remaining vitreoretinal attachments only ceases if the vitre-

Figure 4.2 Dark, annular, glial ring of a posterior vitreous detachment seen in the pupil. Courtesy of Matthew Garston.

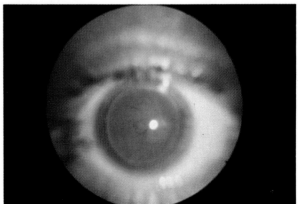

ous ultimately separates from the retina or if the retinal tissue at the site of attachment is pulled free into the vitreous. Adherence of the anterior attachment of the vitreous to the vitreous base may result in the flashing arc of light characteristically seen by patients after a PVD.

Blurred vision may result from large vitreous floaters obscuring the patient's vision, vitreous hemorrhage, or cystoid macular edema (resulting from vitreous strands tugging on the macula). This last finding also produces the symptom of metamorphopsia.

The normal aging process is considered to be the usual mechanism in the production of a PVD; however, trauma can also be responsible for their occurrence. Posterior vitreous detachment has been found to occur in 58% of patients over 50 years of age[5] and in 65% of those between 65 and 85 years of age.[6] It is more likely to be seen in patients who are aphakic or myopic, or have a history of severe ocular trauma or uveitis.

The pathogenesis of a spontaneous PVD appears to be the result of syneresis that produces liquefaction of the vitreous gel and contraction of the fibrous vitreous over the vitreous base. The contraction of collagen fibers over the vitreous base produces an anterior traction on the vitreous that pulls the posterior cortex off of the retina. Liquefaction of the vitreous body allows the vitreous to collapse in an anterior and inferior direction due to gravity (Figure 4.3). This process is enhanced by head trauma, so that even a slight bump on the head may initiate a PVD in older patients.

CLINICAL SIGNIFICANCE

The forward-collapsing motion of the vitreous can exert substantial tractional forces on areas of increased vitreoretinal adhesion, possibly resulting in retinal tears (Figure 4.3). Most of these tears occur anterior to the equator. The frequency of retinal breaks in eyes with a symptomatic PVD has been reported to be between 10% and 15%,[2,3,7] and one study reported that a PVD was found in 80% of eyes with retinal tears.[6]

Retinal tears can be operculated, horseshoe-shaped, or linear (see Chapter 5, page 160). Because of the anterior displacement of the vitreous, the operculum in an operculated tear is generally found anterior to the round tear. The vitreous cortex is usually attached to the flap of a horseshoe tear (Figure 4.3) and the anterior margin of a linear tear. If a small amount of cortex is still attached to the posterior margins of a horseshoe or linear tear, the edges may become rolled due to contraction. A linear tear often occurs along the posterior margin and rarely the anterior margin of lattice degeneration after a PVD. Vitreous strands are attached to the posterior and anterior margins of lattice degeneration (see Lattice Degeneration, page 101). The

Figure 4.3 The vitreous has moved forward and collapsed downward, thus producing traction at sites of increased vitreoretinal adhesion and resultant retinal tears.

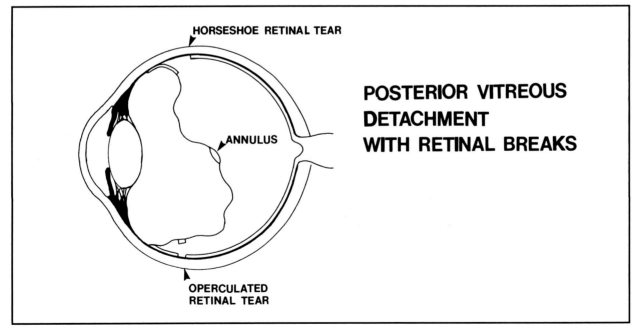

HORSESHOE RETINAL TEAR

ANNULUS

POSTERIOR VITREOUS
DETACHMENT
WITH RETINAL BREAKS

OPERCULATED
RETINAL TEAR

continued vitreous traction on the flap of a retinal tear greatly enhances the chances for the production of a retinal detachment. An operculated retinal tear has a far better prognosis because vitreous traction has been released from its edges. The area of the vitreous base is not involved in a PVD, therefore tears within the base are rare. If they do occur, they are generally secondary to focal areas of strong vitreous attachment such as a zonular traction tuft. Since there is a firm gel structure at the base, the frequency of vitreous liquefaction is low and there is little likelihood of a retinal detachment from a break in the base.[8]

The forward displacement of the vitreous body results in a retrovitreous space that fills with liquefied vitreous. This space can become even larger than that occupied by the collapsing vitreous body. A large reservoir of fluid vitreous is thus made available to pass into any retinal break and result in a retinal detachment.

Another retinal finding associated with a PVD is white-with or -without-pressure, which is the result of vitreous traction[9] (see White-With or -Without-Pressure, page 76.) Another possible finding is edema of the macula and optic disc, which is also produced by traction.[10-12] The edema may disappear if vitreoretinal adhesions are broken, but if the traction exists for a prolonged period of time, irreversible damage can result. Retinal, preretinal, and vitreous hemorrhage can occur after a PVD.[2,13]

REFERENCES

1. Heller MD, Straatsma BR, et al. Detachment of the posterior vitreous in phakic and aphakic eyes. Mod Probl Ophthalmol 1972;10:23.
2. Tasman W. Posterior vitreous detachment and peripheral retinal breaks. Trans Am Acad Ophthalmol Otolaryngol 1968;72:217–224.
3. Jaffe NS. Complications of acute posterior vit-

reous detachment. Arch Ophthalmol 1968; 79:368–371.

4. Moore RF. Subjective "lightning streaks." Br J Ophthalmol 1935;19:545–547.

5. Pischel DK. Detachment of the vitreous as seen with slit-lamp examination. Am J Ophthalmol 1953;36:1497–1507.

6. Tolentino FI, Schepens CL, et al. Vitreoretinal disorders: diagnosis and management. Philadelphia: WB Saunders, 1976;7:130–190.

7. Linder B. Acute posterior vitreous detachment and its retinal complications. A clinical biomicroscopic study. Acta Ophthalmol [Suppl] (Copenh) 1966;87:65–68.

8. Straatsma BR, Foos RY, et al. Rhegmatogenous retinal detachment. In: Duane TD, Jaeger EA, eds. Clinical ophthalmology, vol. 3. Philadelphia: Harper & Row, 1980;27:1–10.

9. Wadsworth JAC. Symposium: retinal detachment. Etiology and pathology. Trans Am Acad Ophthalmol Otolaryngol 1952;56:370–397.

10. Schepens CL. Clinical aspects of pathological changes in the vitreous body. Am J Ophthalmol 1954;38:8–21.

11. Tolentino F, Schepens CL. Edema of posterior pole after cataract extraction. Arch Ophthalmol 1965;74:781–786.

12. Jaffe NS. Vitreous traction of the posterior pole of the fundus due to alterations in the posterior vitreous. Trans Am Acad Ophthalmol Otolaryngol 1967;71:642–652.

13. DeVries S. Retinal hemorrhages in posterior vitreous detachment. Ophthalmologica (Basel) 1951;122:245–248.

Vitreous
Hemorrhage

Figure 4.4 Vitreous hemorrhage is in the center of the photograph and a vitreous strand is at the edge. Symptom would be the sudden onset of many tiny black floaters.

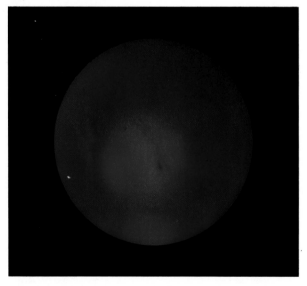

CLINICAL DESCRIPTION

Symptoms of a vitreous bleed are the sudden onset of numerous tiny black floaters—so-called swarm of gnats—that are best seen against a bright background. They are the result of the shadow cast by red blood cells close to the retinal surface. The patient may complain about blurry or smokey vision if a substantial amount of blood is found in the visual axis of the vitreous body (Figure 4.4). If there is a large vitreous hemorrhage, the patient may complain of red vision. Vitreous hemorrhage may occur as the result of trauma or retinal tear, or from any type of hemorrhagic retinopathy (especially diabetes).

A vitreous hemorrhage can also lead to vitreous gel degeneration, which is believed to be the result of the effects of the degenerating red blood cells on the hyaluronic acid present in the vitreous. The result is extensive loss of water from the vitreous gel. Lysis of red blood cells in the vitreous can result in the formation of vitreous membranes. Both of these degenerative changes can produce substantial tractional forces that result in a retinal break or detachment.[1,2]

Blood in the vitreous settles inferiorly due to gravity, where it clots and loses its red pigmentation over several months. Sometimes patients are placed on strict bedrest and bilateral eye patching to reduce head and eye movements to facilitate this gravitational effect. The areas of clotted blood become yellowish white with time and remain stationary in the formed vitreous (Figures 4.5 and 4.6). The clinical finding of yellowish white strands with blood clots intermixed within them is fairly pathognomonic for a previous vitreal bleed.

A pseudomembrane of the vitreous can result from the sheetlike formation of hazy vitreous secondary to vitreous hemorrhage. This pseudomembrane can be mistaken for a retinal detachment. Also, small fresh blood clots in the vitreous close to the retina are bright red and can be mistaken for a retinal break. These two entities are usually differentiated on careful examination by binocular indirect ophthalmoscopy.

CLINICAL SIGNIFICANCE

Repeated vitreous hemorrhages can produce extensive vitreous scarring and degeneration. This often results in vision restricted to hand motion and light perception. Treatment for scarred vitreous is vitrectomy with irrigation and infusion.

REFERENCES

1. Tolentino FT, Schepens CL, et al. Vitreoretinal disorders: diagnosis and management. Philadelphia: WB Saunders, 1976.
2. Pischel DK. Retinal detachment: a manual. Trans Am Acad Ophthalmol Otolaryngol 1965:77.

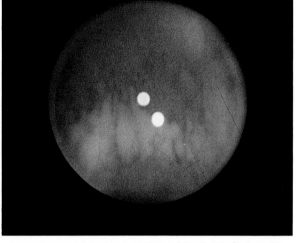

Figure 4.5   Old vitreous bleed in the inferior vitreous is seen as whitish deposits through the indirect condensing lens.

Figure 4.6   B-scan ultrasonography of blood clots scattered in the anterior inferior vitreous.

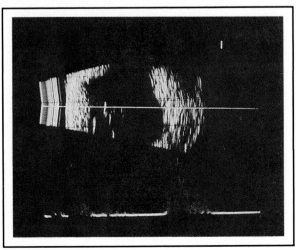

Vitreous Bands and Membranes

Figure 4.7 Vitreous traction band over the superior peripheral retina; each end was anchored to the pars plana. View is through the indirect condensing lens.

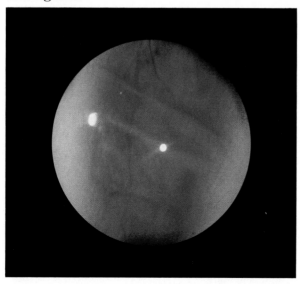

Vitreous bands and membranes appear to be different physical manifestations of the same degenerative process of the vitreous.

CLINICAL DESCRIPTION

They are usually the result of condensation of vitreous gel into strands of sheetlike structures that vary in length, width, thickness, and location. They can be fairly transparent (Figure 4.7) or opaque (Figure 4.8). The membranes can become dense enough to decrease vision markedly. Generally, their construction is that of an acellular hyaline layer with cells that often resemble fibrocytes coating it.[1,2]

Vitreous membranes are usually found over the vitreous base but they can crisscross the vitreous body in any direction. They can be free floating in the liquefied vitreous with each end terminating within the vitreous, or one end may be attached to the retina or pars plana; rarely, both ends are attached. They are more frequently found in myopes and aphakes, and in eyes with vitreoretinal degeneration. Their etiology may be congenital or acquired, as seen in cases of penetrating ocular trauma, vitreous hemorrhage, postinflammatory chorioretinitis, posterior vitreous detachment, and occasionally, retinal neovascularization.[3]

CLINICAL SIGNIFICANCE

Vitreous membranes that have a broad attachment to the retina usually do not produce a retinal break unless considerable force is applied. If such a force occurs, as with ocular trauma, a giant retinal tear may develop. A small area of vitreous attachment requires much less force to produce a retinal break, which usually takes the form of a linear, horseshoe or operculated tear. A sign of traction is the observance of taut membranes that may display stress lines. Other signs suggesting tractional forces are vitreous gel shrinkage and hemorrhage. Some membranes attached to the retina may appear to be lax and gently sway in the vitreous cavity. These may give a false estimation of their tractional forces, because on eye movements, there may be a sudden stretching and abrupt tugging on the underlying retina.

Vitreous membranes may be attached to retinal tufts and meridional folds and traction may result in avulsed pieces of these structures being pulled up into the vitreous (see Figure 3.32). Lattice degeneration, chorioretinal scars, and pigment clumps typically have associated vitreous membranes, and traction may lead to the production of a retinal break (see Lattice Degeneration, Chorioretinal Scar, and Pigment Clumping, pages 101, 120, and 39).

Other signs of exaggerated tractional forces being applied by vitreous membranes or bands

Figure 4.8 Vitreous strand above the inferior peripheral retina seen through the indirect condensing lens (arrow).

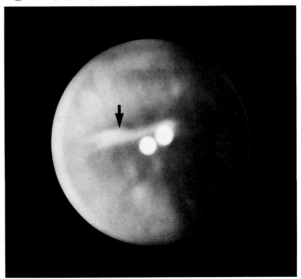

cavity and is frequently twisted like a garland[2] (Figures 4.9 and 4.10). It may or may not be associated with a retinal dialysis or peripheral retinal breaks, and is most frequently seen superonasally, which is the same region in which traumatic retinal dialyses usually occur. It commonly occurs in young people. Inner retinal layers may be stripped away and adherent to the avulsed vitreous base.

CLINICAL SIGNIFICANCE

The existence of an avulsed vitreous base confirms prior trauma. Of itself, it has no clinical significance, except as a cause of sympto-

Figure 4.10 Avulsed vitreous base has been torn free from the region of the ora serrata and is floating in the vitreous. It is common to find twists in the avulsed band that give it a garland appearance.

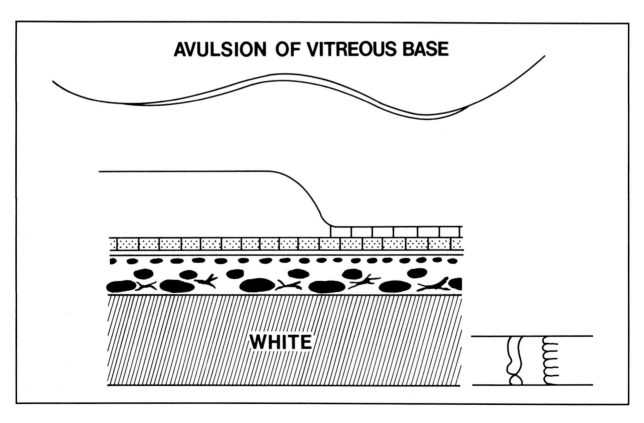

matic floaters. Its clinical significance is in its association with blunt trauma and may therefore be seen in conjunction with vitreous hemorrhage, retinal tears, or retinal detachment. Simultaneous retinal dialysis and avulsion of the vitreous base are found in about 25% of patients with retinal detachment secondary to ocular contusion.[3] Ocular trauma that is not severe enough to produce a retinal tear or avulsion of the vitreous base may result in a tenting-up of the peripheral retina and epithelium of the pars plana. Treatment is not necessary for an avulsed vitreous base.

REFERENCES

1. Teng CC, Chi HH. Vitreous changes and the mechanism of retinal detachment. Am J Ophthalmol 1957;44:335–356.
2. Tasman W. The vitreous. In: Duane TD, Jaeger EA, eds. Clinical ophthalmology, vol. 3. Philadelphia: Harper & Row, 1976;38:14–16.
3. Schepens CL. Retinal detachment and allied diseases. Philadelphia: WB Saunders 1983;5:73.

5 Peripheral Retinal Breaks

CLINICAL DESCRIPTION

A retinal break is a full-thickness break or loss of the sensory retina and is classified as either a hole or a tear. There can also be an incomplete break that involves the inner retinal layers; it is called a retinal excavation, pit, or erosion. The prevalence of retinal breaks ranges from 4% to 18%. They commonly occur in the temporal half of the fundus.[1-6] Full-thickness retinal tears (excluding those at the ora serrata) have been found in 1.9% of autopsied eyes and were bilateral in 11.2% of patients. They are generally located temporally (58%) and inferior (54%); and 95% of most tears are juxtabasal or extrabasal (basal refers to the vitreous base).[7] A study of 1,700 virtually asymptomatic patients revealed that 98 (5.8%) had one or more retinal breaks, nearly all were asymptomatic, and two complained of flashing lights or floaters. Out of the 156 breaks discovered, 120 were holes, 20 were operculated tears, and 16 were horseshoe tears.[8]

Retinal breaks are nearly always found in the peripheral retina due to the existence of strong vitreoretinal adhesion found in this region. The posterior pole rarely has retinal breaks because of the lack of strong vitreoretinal adhesions and a thicker retina supported by numerous large retinal vessels and nerve fibers. Retinal breaks are often referred to as equatorial or oral, based upon their physical location in the fundus. Equatorial breaks are prevalent in older patients and are usually the result of traction on sites of increased vitreoretinal adhesion. Ora breaks are more frequently seen in younger patients and are often the result of ocular trauma.

A retinal hole is a break that is not caused by traction. It is most likely produced by an atrophic process and is generally considered to be the result of underlying vascular disease insufficiency of the choroid and choriocapillaris. Retinal tears are also caused by degeneration of the inner retinal layers, overlying vitreous degeneration, and traction. These tears may be round, linear, or horseshoe-shaped depending on the physical characteristics of the vitreous traction that produced them.

Retinal holes and tears appear red because of the absence of retinal tissue that normally mutes the choroidal reflex. They may be a red to light gray when seen in a detached retina. Retroillumination of a break in a detached retina results in a glowing defect, whereas a retinal hemorrhage appears darker. Often it is necessary to differentiate between a break and a hemorrhage, and this is accomplished by rolling the suspected area with a scleral depressor. A break tends to change color (from dark gray to red) during depression, but a hemorrhage does not. Also, the edges of a retinal break can be seen during scleral depression, but a hemorrhage rolls evenly without displaying elevated edges.

Symptoms of a retinal break include photopsia from vitreous traction, which results from mechanical stimulation to the retina. The flashing lights may be a transient event at the time of the actual formation of the break or continual and episodic due to remaining vitreous adhesion and traction to a torn retinal flap (see Figure 5.11). Flashing lights do not necessarily indicate the production of a retinal break. They may just be the result of vitreous traction that is not sufficient to produce a break, or they occur because the vitreoretinal adhesions were not strong and

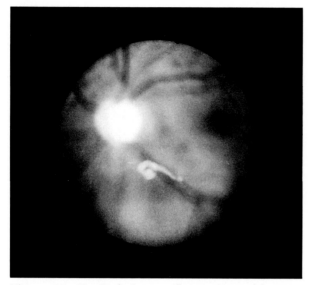

Figure 5.1 Typical vitreous floater. It would cause the symptom of a single floater that moves in the same direction as the eye moves and probably has been noticed for months to years.

vitreous separation occurred without tearing the retina. All of these mechanisms are most frequently associated with advanced vitreous degeneration and posterior vitreous detachment (see Posterior Vitreous Detachment, page 132).

Another symptom is the sudden onset of numerous tiny black floaters, sometimes referred to as a swarm of gnats, in the patient's vision. These are most noticeable when the patient looks at blue sky or a blank white wall. The floaters generally originate in one region of the visual field and slowly spread over most of the other areas of vision. They are the result of small vitreous hemorrhage caused by the rupturing of a retinal blood vessel during the formation of the retinal tear (see Figures 4.4 and 5.9).[9] As long as there is no recurrent bleeding, they slowly disappear over a few days due to the degeneration of red blood cells in the vitreous. This symptom is not to be confused with the patient's complaint of a floater that has been seen for years and moves in the same direction as the eye moves. This is a typical floater that is usually formed from condensed vitreous (Figure 5.1). Sometimes a massive vitreous hemorrhage will obscure a retinal tear. In such cases, B-scan ultrasonography may be able to detect a large retinal tear, but small tears are not detectable with this method.

Any patient who complains of symptoms of photopsia and/or sudden onset of numerous dark floaters should have a retinal examination with a binocular indirect ophthalmoscope through a dilated pupil. If a retinal break is discovered, the fundus examination should be continued to identify additional breaks, because it is not uncommon to find more than one in an eye. There is a report of as many as 29 retinal breaks in one eye.[10] If no retinal break is discovered but a posterior vitreous detachment is present, a follow-up retinal examination is advisable in six months to check for the possible subsequent formation of a retinal break.

A single break was found in about 30% of eyes with a nontraumatic or subclinical retinal detachment, and multiple breaks were found in 70% of these eyes. In eyes with silent breaks, a single break was found in 87.5%. One-half of silent breaks in normal eyes occur in patients less than 40 years old. Yet over 75% of unilateral nontraumatic retinal detachments occur in patients over 40 years of age; therefore it is generally safe to watch a single round hole in the far peripheral retina in patients less than 40 years of age.[9] A retinal break accompanied by symptoms is almost always produced by vitreous traction and has a 30% to 40% chance of developing a retinal detachment.[11,12] Symptomatic breaks are generally treated but sometimes they may simply be watched. The decision whether or not to treat depends upon the medical and ocular status of the patient and the family history.

REFERENCES

1. Adams ST. Retinal breaks in eye bank eyes. Arch Ophthalmol 1956;55:254–260.
2. Okun E. Gross and microscopic pathology in autopsied eyes. III. Retinal breaks without detachment. Am J Ophthalmol 1961;51:369–391.
3. Rutnin U, Schepens CL. Fundus appearance in normal eyes. IV. Retinal breaks and other findings. Am J Ophthalmol 1967;64:1063–1078.
4. Barisak YR, Stein R. Retinal breaks without retinal detachment in autopsied eyes. Acta Ophthalmol (Copenh) 1972;50:147–158.
5. Foos RY. Pastoral peripheral retinal tears. Ann Ophthalmol 1977;6:679–687.
6. Halpern JL. Routine screening of the retinal periphery. Am J Ophthalmol 1966;62:99–102.
7. Straatsma BR, Foos RY, et al. Degenerative diseases of the peripheral retina. In: Duane TD, Jaeger EA, eds. Clinical ophthalmology, vol. 3. Philadelphia: Harper & Row, 1980;26:25–27.
8. Beyer NE. Clinical study of retinal breaks. Trans Am Acad Ophthalmol Otolaryngol 1967;71:461–472.

9. Schepens CL. Retinal detachment and allied diseases. Philadelphia: WB Saunders, 1983:668–672.

10. Pischel. Retinal detachment: a manual. Am Acad Ophthalmol Otolaryngol 1965:73.

11. Davis MD. Natural history of retinal breaks without detachment. Arch Ophthalmol 1974; 92:183–194.

12. Beyer NE. Prognosis of asymptomatic retinal breaks. Arch Ophthalmol 1974;92:208–210.

Retinal Hole

A retinal hole is a retinal break that is not caused by traction and is most likely produced by an atrophic process. It is generally considered to be the result of underlying vascular insufficiency of the choroid and choriocapillaris.

CLINICAL DESCRIPTION

The resultant retinal thinning and degeneration eventually lead to a circumscribed disappearance of the retina, which clinically appears as a hole. These lesions are small, round, red defects typically found in an area of thin and partially opaque retina (Figures 2.10 and 5.2). Their size generally varies from a pinpoint to 1.5 disc diameters.[1] The red color is the result of the absence of the overlying retinal tissue, which allows the red choroidal reflex to appear brighter. They are red to light gray when seen in a detached retina. Retinal holes are generally

Figure 5.2   Three atrophic retina holes in the nasal retina seen through the indirect condensing lens.

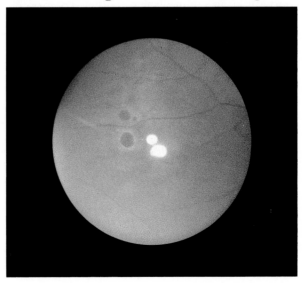

confined to the region between the equator and the ora serrata. Retinal breaks in general most frequently occur in the temporal half of the retina.

HISTOPATHOLOGY

A retinal hole is produced by the loss of retinal tissue in a circumscribed area of thinning. The edges of the hole become rounded with time due to degeneration and contraction (Figure 5.3).

CLINICAL SIGNIFICANCE

Most retinal holes do not lead to a retinal detachment because there is no strong vitreous traction present. They should be followed on a periodic basis, however, to rule out the formation of a subclinical retinal detachment. An atrophic hole has a 7% chance of progressing into a retinal detachment.[2] If such a detachment should occur, treatment with cryotherapy or photocoagulation may be indicated.

Figure 5.3 Retinal hole shows the loss of the sensory retina, thus allowing the choriocapillaris to be seen more readily. This is why retinal holes look redder than the surrounding fundus. Their edges are rounded due to degeneration and contraction.

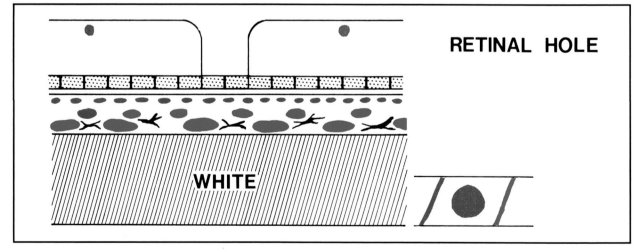

REFERENCES

1. Schepens CL. Retinal detachment and allied diseases. Philadelphia: WB Saunders, 1983:158.
2. Davis MD. Natural history of retinal breaks without detachment. Arch Ophthalmol 1974; 92:183–194.

Operculated Retinal Tear

CLINICAL DESCRIPTION

Operculated retinal tears are round, red holes with the avulsed round retinal plug (operculum) adherent to the detached cortical vitreous (see Figure 5.6). The operculum is seen floating in the vitreous cavity (see Figure 2.10) and is frequently located anterior to the hole. This is due to the anterior displacement of the vitreous during a posterior vitreous detachment and collapse (see Figure 4.3). However, the operculum can be found directly above the hole or in any direction from the hole, depending on the force of vitreous traction at the time of avulsion. The operculum usually appears smaller than the hole from which it came, which is secondary to degeneration and contraction due to the loss of blood supply to the avulsed retinal tissue.

Operculated tears are usually located between the ora serrata and the equator, generally in the temporal half of the fundus. They frequently occur in areas of lattice degeneration and thinning. The holes may have small yellow spheroids within their borders. These are known as pathologic drusen (Figures 5.4 and 5.5) and are the result of giant drusen formation by the pigment epithelium in response to their abnormal condition of no overlying sensory retina.[1]

The holes may be surrounded by white-with or -without-pressure (see Figure 3.49). Therefore, it is advisable that scleral depression be performed in an area of the fundus where a round floater is found in the vitreous. This may enhance the appearance of a retinal break that is just barely visible (see White-With or -Without-Pressure, page 76). Circumscribed subretinal fluid may accumulate around the hole, producing a subclinical or localized retinal detachment (Figure 5.4). If the subclinical retinal detachment remains stationary for three months or longer, a pigmented retinal demarcation line may be produced (Figure 5.5). This pigment line is produced by the proliferation of pigment epithelial cells and is believed to form a weak bond at the edge of the retinal detachment that may retard its progression (see Chapter 6).

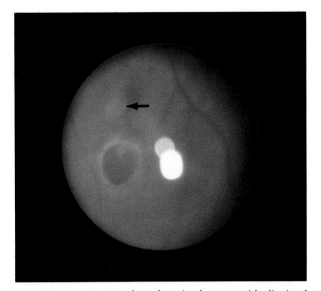

Figure 5.4 Operculated retinal tear with limited surrounding retinal detachment, a large drusen at the edge of its base, and the operculum floating above (arrow) still attached to the detached vitreous. View is through the indirect condensing lens.

HISTOPATHOLOGY

The avulsed retinal tissue that is attached to the cortical vitreous displays marked degeneration and contraction with time. The retinal hole shows full-thickness loss of sensory retina,

Figure 5.5 Operculated retinal tear with surrounding limited retinal detachment that remained stationary long enough to produce a pigmented demarcation line. There are large drusen underneath the detached retina, and the operculum can be seen above the tear still attached to the detached vitreous. View is of the inferior nasal retina through the indirect condensing lens.

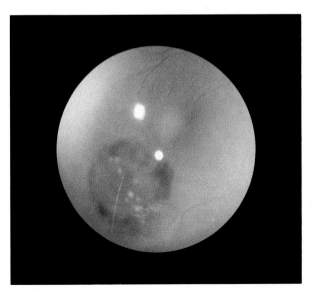

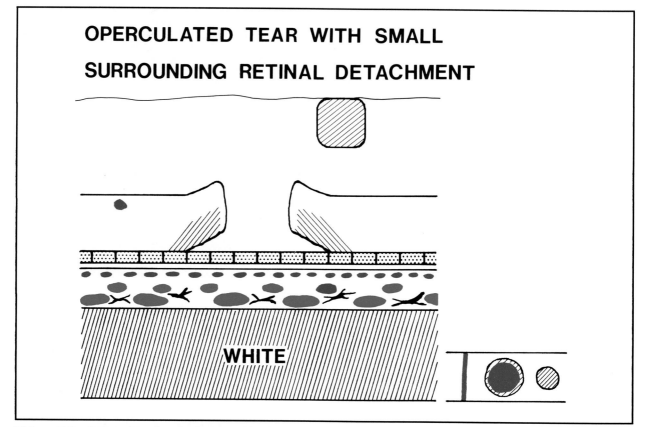

OPERCULATED TEAR WITH SMALL SURROUNDING RETINAL DETACHMENT

WHITE

Figure 5.6 Operculated retinal tear with operculum still attached to the detached vitreous and a limited surrounding retinal detachment, which gives the tear a white collar. The operculum is smaller than the retinal break due to degeneration and contraction, which are also responsible for the rounded edges of the break.

leaving the pigment epithelium in place (Figure 5.6). Surrounding the hole may be an accumulation of liquefied vitreous in the subneural space, resulting in a subclinical retinal detachment.

CLINICAL SIGNIFICANCE

Operculated retinal tears can lead to a clinically significant retinal detachment. The risk of retinal separation from an operculated tear is much less than the risk from a horseshoe tear because vitreous traction to the retina has been released. There may be an associated vitreous hemorrhage if a retinal vessel traversing the involved area is ruptured during formation of the tear.

No treatment is necessary for asymptomatic operculated tears without detachment unless they occur in the presence of high myopia, aphakia, extensive vitreoretinal degeneration, or family or personal history of retinal detachment. Symptomatic tears, especially those with localized retinal detachment, may be adequately treated with cryotherapy or photocoagulation (Figures 5.7 and 5.8).

REFERENCE

1. Smiddy WE, Green RW. Retinal dialysis: pathology and pathogenesis. Retina 1982;2:94–116.

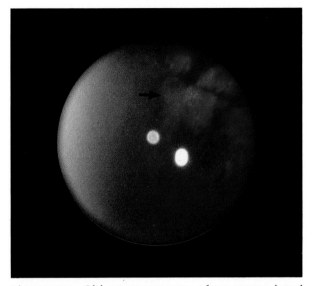

Figure 5.7 Old cryopexy scar of an operculated tear seen through an indirect condensing lens. Note circular operculum above the lesion still attached to the detached vitreous (arrow).

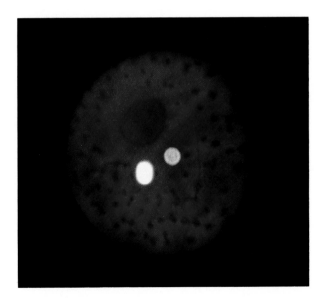

Figure 5.8 Rows of argon laser photocoagulation around an operculated retina tear seen through the indirect condensing lens.

Horseshoe or
Linear Retinal Tear

A horseshoe or linear retinal tear is the result of vitreous traction to an area of thinned or atrophic retina. This frequently affects areas of the retina that suffer from lattice degeneration.

CLINICAL DESCRIPTION

As the vitreous separates from the retina and undergoes collapse, tractional forces are ap-

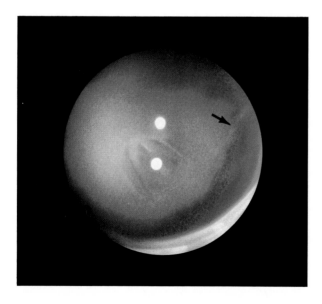

Figure 5.9 Horseshoe retinal tear in a retinal detachment seen through the indirect condensing lens. Note the retinal hemorrhage on either side of the base of the flap, the whitish color of the detached retina, and loss of choroidal pattern beneath the detachment. Note also that the retinal tear stopped its anterior progress at the posterior border of the vitreous base, which is seen as a faint white line on the detached retina (arrow).

plied to areas of tight vitreoretinal adherence. If the traction is sufficient, it may tear a flap of retina, with the anterior margin remaining continuous with the peripheral retina (see Figure 4.3). As the vitreous moves forward, the flap assumes a horseshoe or linear shape; in a horseshoe tear, the apex points toward the posterior pole (Figures 2.10 and 5.9). Sometimes strands of retinal tissue can be seen bridging the break from the flap to the edge of the tear (Figure 5.10).

The tear itself appears red due to the loss of retinal tissue that normally mutes the choroidal reflex; however, it has a red to a light gray color in detached retinas. The flap appears whitish because of the edema and subsequent degeneration resulting from the loss of circulation to the outer retinal layers and sometimes to the inner retinal layers from the choriocapillaris and retinal circulation respectively (Figure 5.11). Over time, the flap shrinks in size as the tissue degenerates and contracts (Figures 2.10 and 5.12). Sometimes the retinal flap takes unusual shapes, like an hourglass or J-shape, which can be the result of a retinal blood vessel coursing over the flap.

Horseshoe or linear tears can be located in any part of the peripheral retina. They commonly occur at the posterior border of the vitreous base, areas of lattice degeneration, pigment clumps, or retinal tufts (see Figure 3.70). These tears are sometimes associated with a chorioretinal scar (Figure 5.10).

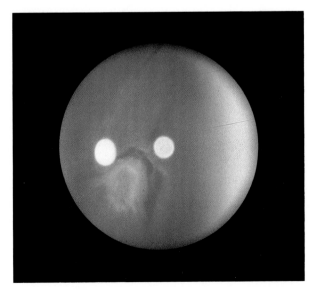

Figure 5.10 Horseshoe retinal tear in a retinal detachment in the superior temporal fundus seen through the indirect condensing lens. The tear was probably produced by vitreous traction on a chorioretinal scar seen on the flap. Note that there are still some strands of retinal tissue bridging the gap of the break. The retinal detachment looks whitish and there is loss of underlying choroidal detail.

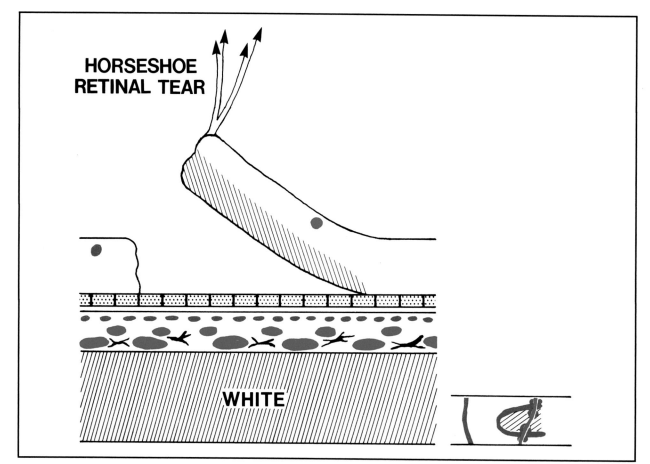

Figure 5.11 Horseshoe retinal tear with vitreous traction. The shearing of a retinal venule has resulted in vitreous and retinal hemorrhage. The flap appears whitish due to degeneration from the loss of apposition to the choriocapillaris. The flap is a little smaller than the break due to degeneration and contraction, which is also responsible for the rounded edges of the break.

HISTOPATHOLOGY

The histopathology of a horseshoe or linear tear is similar to that of an operculated tear. It is characterized by thinning and atrophy of the retinal layers with organized vitreous strands attached to its borders (Figure 5.12).

CLINICAL SIGNIFICANCE

Horseshoe or linear tears are the leading cause of rhegmatogenous retinal detachment. A symptomatic horseshoe tear has a 30% chance of progressing to a retinal detachment[1]; adhesion of the remaining vitreous to the flap allows for continued tractional forces, which greatly increase the chances for the production of a retinal detachment. Sometimes the vitreous strands to a retinal flap can be readily seen (Figure 2.10). There is some evidence to suggest that intrabasal tears are at low risk to develop a clinical retinal detachment.[2] They are more common in eyes with myopia, lattice degeneration, peripheral retinal degeneration, and aphakia. They frequently appear at the vitreous base where there is a sharp or irregular posterior margin. Their frequency increases with age, suggesting that they are degenerative in nature. Vitreous hemorrhage is a frequent concomitant finding and is the result of tearing of a retinal vessel that bridges the tear (see Figures 4.4 and 5.9) (see Vitreous Hemorrhage, page 138). Premonitory symptoms are light flashes, recent floaters, and a progressive loss of peripheral vision if a retinal detachment is produced.

Asymptomatic horseshoe or linear tears are generally treated due to their propensity to produce retinal detachments. Symptomatic tears without detachment are always treated, usually with cryopexy or photocoagulation. In the presence of retinal detachment, scleral buckling procedures are indicated.

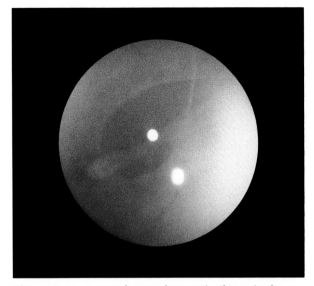

Figure 5.12 Large horseshoe retinal tear in the superior temporal retina seen through the indirect condensing lens. Note that the flap is markedly narrower than the break it came from, indicating a long-standing condition. There was no retinal detachment associated with the tear, which probably indicates the absence of liquefied vitreous above the break.

REFERENCES

1. Davis MD. Natural history of retinal breaks without detachment. Arch Ophthalmol 1974; 92:183–194.
2. Sigelman J. Vitreous base classification of retinal tears: clinical application. Surv Ophthalmol 1980;25:59–74.

Retinal Dialysis

CLINICAL DESCRIPTION

A retinal dialysis is a retinal tear that occurs at the ora serrata and is concentric with the ora (Figure 5.13). Most tears are less than 90 degrees and they may occur bilaterally. The choroidal pattern becomes more visible in the area of the dialysis due to the loss of overlying retinal tissue (Figure 5.14). If the edge of the dialysis remains close to the underlying choroid, the break may not be discovered until scleral depression is performed. The condition is often

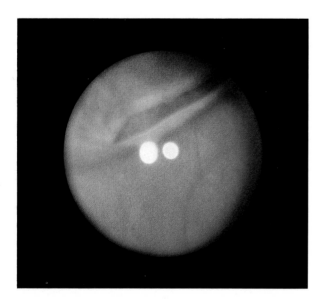

Figure 5.13 Superior edge of posttraumatic retinal dialysis in the superior nasal fundus seen through the indirect condensing lens during scleral depression. Note that there is a small rim of detached retinal tissue just posterior to the ora serrata, followed by the dialysis, which allows a view of the choroid. There is another small rim of detached retina on the posterior aspect of the dialysis.

Treatme
buckling with
erally favorab

REFERENCE

1. Schepens
   diseases.
   10:90–91
2. Anderson
   disinserti
   J Ophthal
3. Smiddy '
   thology a
4. Dobbie J(
   rata and
   retinal d
   68:610–6
5. Syrdalen
   Acta Oph
6. Weidenth
   dus chan
   Am J Opl

asymptomatic, with a slowly progressive retinal detachment that is often characterized by successive demarcation lines. It may represent an exaggerated coalescence of peripheral cytoid degeneration or retinoschisis. In a true dialysis, the posterior border of the vitreous base coincides with the ora serrata. If the posterior border lies slightly posterior to the ora serrata, a skirt of retinal tissue remains attached to the ora. Both of these are usually regarded as retinal ora dialyses,[1] but some consider the latter to be retinal tears instead of true dialyses. As the vitreous contracts, the tears become more elevated in conjunction with increasing retinal detachment. Males are more frequently affected than females.

HISTOPATHOLOGY

The retina is separated at or just posterior to the ora serrata (Figure 5.15).[2,3] The retina itself may appear normal or dysplastic. The overlying vitreous is usually normal in appearance, without liquefaction.

CLINICAL SIGNIFICANCE

Inferotemporal retinal dialysis of the young is a spontaneous dialysis associated with an asymptomatic, slowly progressive retinal detachment that is often associated with multiple demarcation lines.[4] Males are more frequently affected than females and its bilaterality stands in marked contrast to traumatic retinal dialyses.

Traumatic retinal dialyses are more commonly found superonasal and are unilateral[5]; however, a blow to the eye from an angle to the temporal limbus can result in an inferior, temporally located dialysis.[6] The condition may be associated with vitreous hemorrhage and other stigmata of eye trauma. A traumatic dialysis may

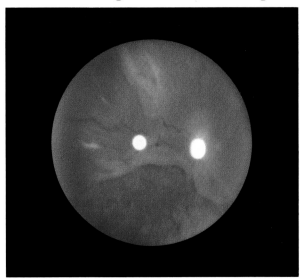

Figure 5.14 Retinal dialysis after vitrectomy for scarred vitreous in a patient with diabetic eye disease. Note whitish detached retina with folds and unobstructed view of brownish-appearing choroid just anterior to retinal detachment. View is of the inferior retina through an indirect condensing lens.

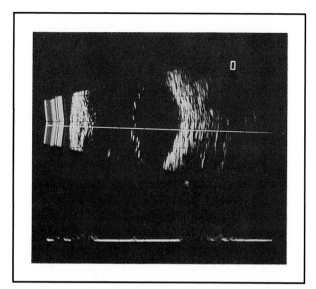

Figure 6.6 B-scan ultrasonogram of bullous retinal detachment into the middle of the vitreous cavity. Note the folds in the detached retina. White striated area on the left is feedback noise from the closed eyelid to the transducer.

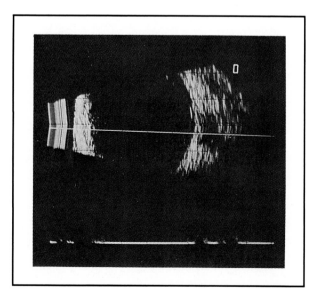

Figure 6.7 B-scan ultrasonogram of a shallow retinal detachment just barely detached from the posterior region of the globe.

entiating among macular cyst, partial macular break, and full-thickness hole is difficult. High magnification with a biomicroscope and contact lens or Hruby lens is usually required to detect a macular cyst. Rupture of the inner wall of a cyst will not result in a retinal detachment if the outer wall is intact. Only a full-thickness break results in a retinal detachment. True full-thickness macular holes were present in only 0.62% of 5,442 cases of retinal detachment.[2]

The finding of numerous brown specks in the anterior vitreous during biomicroscopy strongly suggests a retinal break with associated retinal detachment (Figure 6.9). These specks represent free-floating RPE cells[3] and are commonly referred to as "tobacco dust" or Shaffer's sign of the vitreous. Mild anterior uveitis is often associated with a retinal detachment; therefore biomicroscopy can be useful in its diagnosis.

A careful evaluation of the retina with indirect ophthalmoscopy and Goldmann contact lens should be carried out to locate and identify all the retinal breaks associated with the detachment. These breaks are usually found in the far periphery of the retina in the region of the vitreous base. They frequently occur in areas of lattice degeneration (see Figures 3.69, 3.70, and 3.71) or in hyperpigmented areas that are the locus of firm vitreoretinal adhesions (see Figure 3.15). Old chorioretinal scars (see Figure 3.78) should also be carefully examined for retinal breaks that occur at the edges of the scar. If none is found, a nonrhegmatogenous retinal detachment must be suspected.

Figure 6.8 A large posttraumatic macular hole with a small surrounding localized retinal detachment. Note the surrounding chorioretinal atrophy with pigment proliferation and migration.

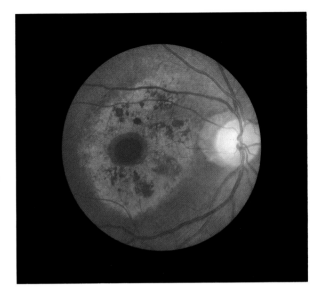

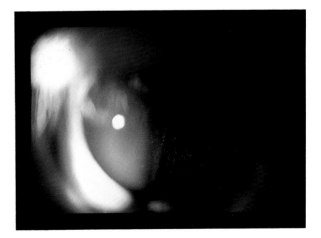

Figure 6.9 "Tobacco dust" (pigment cells) in the anterior vitreous seen during biomicroscopy of a patient with a retinal detachment.

ment in one eye greatly enhances the risk for the fellow eye. Family history is very important, as persons with hereditary diseases such as Wagner's disease (see Wagner's Hereditary Vitreoretinal Degeneration, page 116) and high myopia are more likely to develop a retinal detachment. Patients with vitreal and retinal diseases are at substantial risk; it is helpful to note that approximately 50% of rhegmatogenous retinal detachments are caused by retinal tears demonstrating vitreous traction, about 30% are associated with lattice degeneration, and approximately 20% are the result of retinal dialyses or holes.[20,21] Another study reported that symptomatic retinal tears account for 30% to 50% of rhegmatogenous retinal detachments and asymptomatic breaks only account for 10%.[11]

The speed at which a retinal detachment progresses toward the posterior pole mainly depends on the number and size of the breaks, their distance from the posterior pole, and the degree of preretinal organization. A detachment from equatorial breaks usually involves the posterior pole sooner than one from oral breaks.

Location is important in the progression of a detachment. A superiorly located detachment is more likely to progress because gravity facilitates downward movement of the subretinal fluid. The opposite is true of a detachment located in the inferior region of the fundus. A retinal detachment found in the superotemporal quadrant of the fundus is more hazardous to the visual status of the patient because its downward movement can easily result in macular involvement. A superonasal detachment is not as visually threatening, however, because the optic disc acts as an obstruction to macular involvement.

The region of the retina involved in a rhegmatogenous detachment can aid in localizing the retinal break. A detachment that is superior and travels approximately the same distance inferior in the nasal and temporal halves of the fundus probably indicates a break close to the 12 o'clock position. A retinal break at the 6 o'clock position would produce a detachment that would be approximately a mirror image of the one produced by the 12 o'clock break. A retinal detachment that ranged from the superonasal to the inferonasal region to partly into the inferotemporal region would be most indicative of a break in the superonasal region of the fundus. The billowing movement of a retinal detachment studied with an understanding of gravitational forces can facilitate the discovery of retinal breaks.

Once the macula is detached (Figure 6.3), the patient may never reattain full visual acuity. If the macula is off for over a month, the best visual acuity that could be hopefully recovered is 20/70, and over three months of detachment, 20/200 would be the best that could be anticipated. A retina that is totally detached for over two years is not likely to demonstrate visual improvement after reattachment, but some remarkable exceptions have occurred.[6] The preoperative visual acuity can be a prognosis for postoperative acuity. Vision limited to hand motion may still show vast improvement following reattachment; however, in the absence of light perception, no functional recovery is possible. Exceptions are patients with high ocular tension of fairly recent origin associated with retinal detachment and no light perception vision; measurable vision may return after reattachment and lowering of intraocular tension.[6]

A retinal detachment may extend past the ora serrata, causing the nonpigmented epithelium of the pars plana to separate from the pigmented epithelium. This is frequently observed in cases of traumatic retinal dialysis or giant retinal tear (see Retinal Dialysis, page 164, and Giant Retinal Tear, page 168). This can also occur whenever there is marked vitreous traction on the vitreous base and it is frequently seen in massive periretinal proliferation (see

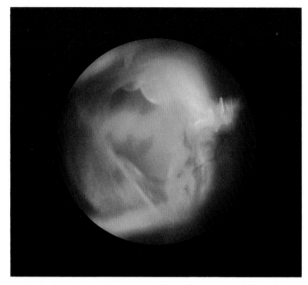

Figure 6.11 Total retinal detachment with a large retinal tear seen in the anterior vitreous cavity during biomicroscopy. Detached retina looks grayish with blood vessels traversing it.

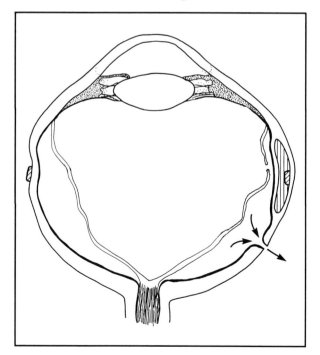

Massive Periretinal Proliferation, page 193). Detached ciliary epithelium is invisible when viewed straight on, but appears as a translucent membrane when seen in profile during scleral depression or on a scleral buckle. Detachment of the ciliary epithelium occurs more often above the horizontal meridian and nasally than below and temporally. The detachment can extend as far anterior as the ciliary processes. The detached ora serrata is seen as a narrow lightly pigmented scalloped zone that separates the transparent ciliary epithelium from the thicker detached retina. A faint pigment line in the underlying choroid denotes where the ora serrata was attached and it has the contour of the ora bays and teeth.[2,6]

Occasionally there is an iatrogenic cause for retinal detachment, for example, after a complicated cataract extraction in which there is vitreous loss and incarceration in the corneoscleral wound. This may lead to an inferior tractional nonrhegmatogenous detachment.[6]

A total retinal detachment results from the separation of the entire sensory retina from the pigment epithelium. This most often occurs in eyes with large retinal breaks (Figure 6.11), especially giant retinal tears or with numerous breaks; however, sometimes a single, small break can produce a total detachment if a large amount of liquefied vitreous is available. Total detachments are more likely to be found in aphakic than phakic eyes.

If the detached retina remains fixed to the ora serrata and the optic disc, it will produce a funnel-shaped structure with the wide end an-

Figure 6.12 Diagram of eye with a total rhegmatogenous retinal detachment. A scleral buckle has been placed in a scleral bed under the retinal break. An encircling band is in place around the globe that fits into a groove in the buckle. A perforation has been made in the globe to evacuate the subretinal fluid.

terior and the disc at the narrow end (Figures 6.12 and 6.13). Usually the optic disc can be seen at the apex of the funnel (Figure 6.14). This whitish funnel-shaped structure is also known as a morning-glory detachment due to its resemblance to the horn-shaped flower. If the detached retina separates from the ora serrata, it will collapse toward the center of the vitreous cavity (Figure 6.15). Both the anatomical and visual prognoses for reattachment of a totally detached retina are poor.

HISTOPATHOLOGY

Sections of detached retinas show fluid accumulation in the subretinal space and degeneration of the photoreceptor layer, and the outer layers of the retina become edematous and atrophic after two to three months of detachment. Microcystoid degeneration is initially seen, followed by coalescence of the cystoid spaces into a larger cyst with time. This microcystoid degeneration causes the honeycomb appearance to the detached retina on clinical examination.[22] Some proliferation of glial and connective tissue occurs and increases with time.

The fluid under a retinal detachment can be seen on histology sections (see Figure 3.14); if no fluid is seen, the retinal separation is artifactual in origin. The characteristics of this fluid can be indicative of the etiology of the detachment; for example, eosinophils are found in a nematode endophthalmitis, foamy macrophages and periodic acid-Schiff (PAS)-positive fluid in Coat's disease, and serous proteinaceous fluid in choroidal tumors.

CLINICAL SIGNIFICANCE

The clinical significance of a rhegmatogenous retinal detachment is that it usually leads

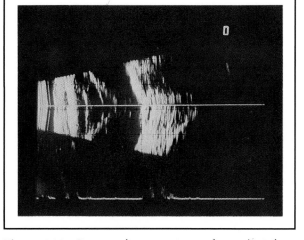

Figure 6.13 B-scan ultrasonogram of morning-glory retinal detachment seen as funnel-shaped structure in the vitreous cavity.

Figure 6.14 Long-standing morning-glory retinal detachment. Note small retinal hemorrhage, white areas of retinal gliosis. Optic disc can be seen at the bottom of the funnel of detached retina in the center of the figure.

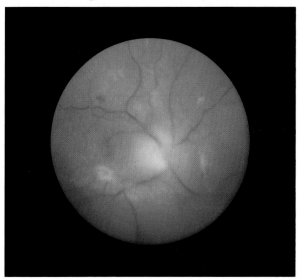

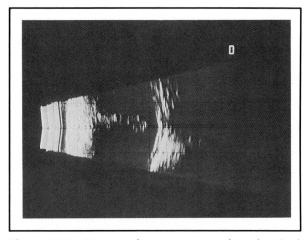

Figure 6.15 B-scan ultrasonogram of total retinal detachment that has collapsed on itself in the center of the vitreous cavity.

to total blindness if not accurately diagnosed and surgically corrected. The significance of a nonrhegmatogenous retinal detachment depends on the underlying pathology. The most worrisome causes are malignant intraocular tumors.

REFERENCES

1. Pischel DK. Retinal detachment: a manual, ed. 2. Am Acad Ophthalmol Otolaryngol 1965;10–85, 197–199.
2. von Pirquet SR, Jaugschaffer O. Treatment of macular holes by photocoagulation. In: Schepens CL, Regan CDJ, eds. Controversial aspects of the management of retinal detachment. Boston: Little, Brown, 1966:181.
3. Machemer R. Massive periretinal proliferation: a logical approach to therapy. Trans Am Ophthalmol Soc 1977;75:556–586.
4. Jones WL. Intraocular metastatic disease to the eye. J Am Optom Assoc 1981;52:741–744.
5. Yanoff M, Fine SF. Ocular pathology; ed 2. Philadelphia: Harper & Row, 1982:461, 563.
6. Schepens CL. Retinal detachment and allied diseases. Philadelphia: WB Saunders, 1983: 69,93,182,212,224.
7. Cox MS, Schepens CL, et al. Traumatic retinal detachment due to ocular contusion. Arch Ophthalmol 1966;76:678–685.
8. Freeman HM, Cox MS, et al. Traumatic retinal detachments. Int Ophthalmol Clin 1974;14:151–170.
9. Ashrafzadeh MT, Schepens CL, et al. Aphakic and phakic retinal detachment. Arch Ophthalmol 1973;89:476–483.
10. Norton EWD. Retinal detachment in aphakia. Am J Ophthalmol 1964;58:111–124.
11. Davis MD. Natural history of retinal breaks without detachment. Arch Ophthalmol 1974; 92:183–194.
12. Wilkes SR, Beard C, et al. The incidence of retinal detachment in Rochester, Minnesota, 1970–1978. Am J Ophthalmol 1982;94:670–673.
13. Tasman W. Retinal detachment in children.

Trans Am Acad Ophthalmol Otolaryngol 1967;71:455–460.

14. Haimann MH, Burton TC, et al. Epidemiology of retinal detachment. Arch Ophthalmol 1982; 100:289–292.

15. Michaelson IC, Stein R. A national study in the prevention of retinal detachment. Ann Ophthalmol 1969;1:49–55.

16. Okun E. Gross and microscopic pathology in autopsied eyes. III. Retinal breaks without detachment. Am J Ophthalmol 1961;51:369–391.

17. Schepens CL, Marden D. Data on the natural history of retinal detachment: further characterization of certain unilateral nontraumatic cases. Am J Ophthalmol 1966;61:213–226.

18. Schepens CL, Marden D. Data on the natural history of retinal detachment. I. Age and sex relationships. Arch Ophthalmol 1961;66:631–642.

19. Amsler M, Schiff-Wertheimer S. Le decollement de la retinae in Traite de ophthalmologie, vol. 5. Bailliart P, eds. Paris: Masson & Cie, 1939:559–576.

20. Beyer NE. The natural history of the retinopathies of retinal detachment and preventive treatment. Isr J Med Sci 1972;8:1417–1420.

21. Straatsma BR, Allen RA. Lattice degeneration of the retina. Trans Am Acad Ophthalmol Otolaryngol 1962;66:600–613.

22. Hogan MJ, Zimmerman LE. Ophthalmic pathology: an atlas and textbook, ed 2. Philadelphia: WB Saunders, 1962:549–569.

Demarcation Lines

CLINICAL DESCRIPTION

A pigmented or gray-white demarcation line (sometimes called a friction line or water mark) is frequently found associated with a retinal detachment, past or present. If an edge of a retinal detachment remains stationary for at least three months, hyperplasia of the pigment epithelium at the detachment margin may occur (Figures 6.16 and 6.17). This is probably the result of mechanical irritation to the border caused by the detachment. The demarcation line

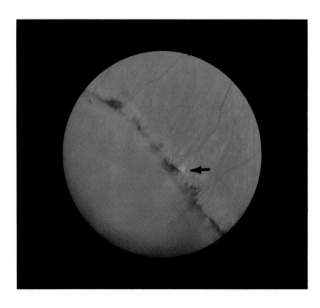

Figure 6.16 Long-standing bullous retinal detachment shows typical pigmented demarcation line at posterior edge and a small area of chorioretinal atrophy (arrow). Note that the detached retina looks whitish and hides the underlying choroidal pattern. This detachment has a taut appearance without any folds present.

Figure 6.17 White demarcation line remains after reattachment of retina.

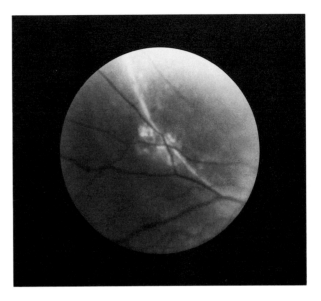

indicates that the detachment has been stationary for at least three months.

The pigmented demarcation line is usually found along the posterior edge of a detachment, just posterior to the border (Figure 6.18). Sometimes the pigmentation is seen as a narrow band on the detachment side of the border. A retinal hole or operculated retinal tear may develop a small surrounding detachment which may have a surrounding pigmented demarcation line, if the detachment is stationary (see Figure 5.5). An

Figure 6.18 Pigmented demarcation line is secondary to pigment epithelial hyperplasia at the edge of the retinal detachment.

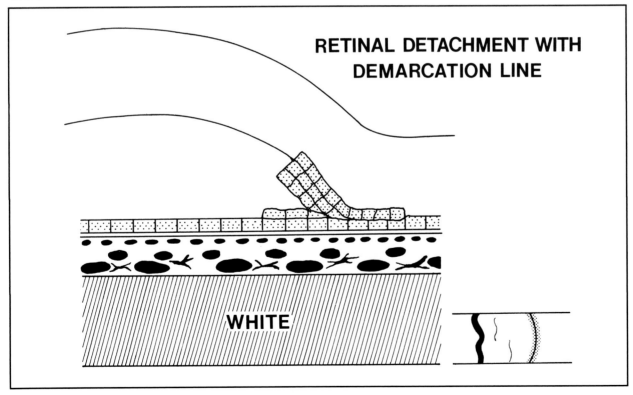

RETINAL DETACHMENT WITH DEMARCATION LINE

WHITE

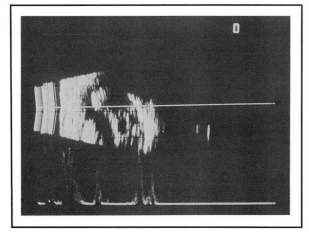

Figure 6.21 B-scan ultrasonogram of a traumatic retinal detachment that has been off for over 40 years. Note the large macrocyst, which is a dark circle in the detached retina in the posterior portion of the vitreous cavity. Anterior aspect of the eye is on the left in the figure.

Figure 6.22 Among the billowing folds of this long-standing retinal detachment there is a macrocyst (arrow). View is through the indirect condensing lens.

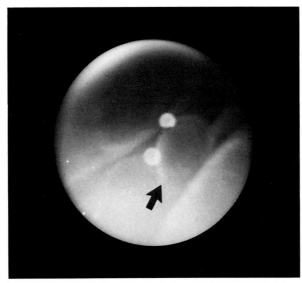

Deep folds may form between bullae which may attach the bullae to each other. The sites of adherence show interruptions of the internal limiting membrane and a proliferation of fibrocytes.[1] Severe fixed folds may produce sharp bends or kinks in the retinal vessels, which may embarrass the existing circulation and result in hemorrhages.

Long-standing detachments often become transparent and thin with time, making it possible to clearly see underlying structures. Also, large macrocysts may develop in the middle layers of the detached retina (Figures 6.21 and 6.22). Other changes seen are reactive pigment proliferation (Figure 6.14), degeneration of the pigment epithelium, thickening of the lamina vitrea, and formation of drusen. The choroid often shows marked degenerative changes and the walls of the vessels of the choriocapillaris become hyalinized.[1] Long-standing detachments have a greater frequency of being totally detached.

CLINICAL SIGNIFICANCE

Often the folding and proliferation of glial tissue seals the retinal breaks on the detached retina, thus trapping the subretinal fluid. Subsequently, macrophages, proliferating pigment cells, cholesterol crystals from small hemorrhages, and other toxic products accumulate to act as irritants and produce secondary uveitis. The uveitis may cause secondary glaucoma, which can eventually lead to enucleation. Hemorrhaging from degenerating retina and choroid is not uncommon and can result in further intraocular inflammation.[1]

REFERENCE

1. Hogan MJ, Zimmerman LE. Ophthalmic pathology: an atlas and textbook, ed 2. Philadelphia: WB Saunders, 1962:549–569.

Massive Periretinal
Proliferation

CLINICAL DESCRIPTION

Massive periretinal proliferation (MPP), also known as massive preretinal retraction (MPR), massive vitreous retraction syndrome, and currently proliferative vitreoretinopathy (PVR), is a malignant form of retinal detachment characterized by large, fixed retinal folds. The folds are usually triangular with rounded corners, and the apex of the triangle is close to the optic disc. Folds can be circular (Figure 6.23) and there may be isolated star-shaped retinal folds (Figure 6.24). Generally, the entire retina

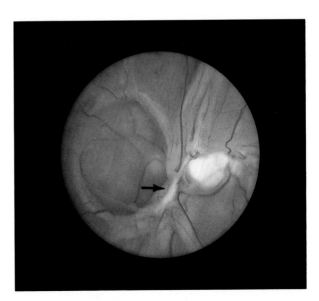

Figure 6.23 Massive periretinal proliferation following retinal detachment surgery in a highly myopic patient. The retina has been pulled off into a circular equatorial fold. Note a fibrotic epiretinal membrane (arrow). Optic disc is bright, white, oval area.

193

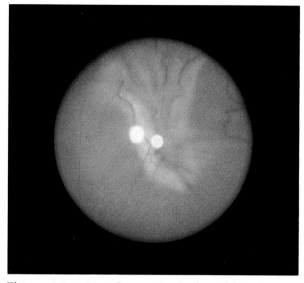

Figure 6.24 Massive periretinal proliferation following retinal detachment surgery in an aphakic patient. View is of the superior nasal fundus through the indirect condensing lens. Note the contraction membrane that has pulled the retina free from the pigment epithelium.

is pulled off, due to contraction of a transvitreal membrane located in the equatorial zone and preretinal membranes. The transvitreal membrane forms across the posterior vitreous face of a posterior vitreous detachment.[1] The RD that forms is a funnel-shaped structure with the narrow end posterior. In the early developmental stages, the optic disc can be seen at the bottom of the funnel but as the process advances, the optic disc is hidden from view with continued collapse of the funnel. Sometimes areas of the fundus previously treated with photocoagulation or cryopexy will not become detached during MPP. Retinal breaks may form at the edge of a previously treated area or at any location in the retina.

Massive preretinal retraction may rarely occur in patients with a rhegmatogenous retinal detachment without previous retinal detachment surgery; however, it is generally seen in patients who have undergone retinal surgery. It is most likely to develop in cases of rhegmatogenous retinal detachment associated with Wagner's vitreoretinal degeneration, lattice retinal degeneration, giant retinal tear, penetrating ocular injury, massive vitreous hemorrhage, and surgical aphakia with vitreous loss. It sometimes occurs in eyes with a nonrhegmatogenous detachment following severe intraocular inflammation.[2]

Onset of MPP is acute and it can produce large areas of retinal detachment overnight; within weeks the process can become well established. The condition seems to occur some 6 to 12 weeks after successful reattachment but in all likelihood, the process was probably ongoing for some time. When sufficient traction has developed, there can be a sudden detachment.[1] Also, when sufficient traction produces a retinal break, the rush of liquified vitreous into the subretinal space can weaken the bond between the photoreceptors and pigment epithelium. This coupled with strong vitreal traction can cause the rapid development of a RD. Early in the development of this process, the fundus reflex changes to a gray color and fundus detail becomes indistinct due to vitreous haze. This haze results from a marked outpouring of serum protein into the vitreous gel and resultant Tyndall effect. Retinal vessels become dilated and tortuous and intraretinal hemorrhages are not unusual, especially at the equator.

Preretinal and equatorial membranes composed of fibrocellular tissue with collagen-like fibers (myofibroblasts) mature, contract, and produce strong tractional forces. The intense traction of these membranes causes the retina to detach and form large retinal folds. Experimental studies suggest that preretinal membranes may be derived from pigment epithelial and glial cells.[3,4] These cells appear to proliferate on the preretinal, retroretinal surfaces and posterior vitreous surface which later contract. Epiremnal membranes are more commonly seen in the inferior fundus.

CLINICAL SIGNIFICANCE

The prognosis for patients with MPP is poor. Retinal detachments frequently recur following a scleral buckling operation, and many become inoperable. Surgery for rhegmatogenous RD is successful in more than 90% of cases and MPP is the most frequent cause of failures.[5]

Treatment requires vitrectomy, scleral buckling with an encircling band, and complete drainage of subretinal fluid to reattach the retina.[4] It is sometimes necessary to inject air, silicone, or sulfur hexafluoride (SF_6) into the vitreous cavity to flatten out the retina against the pigment epithelium. Star-shaped retinal folds should be included onto the buckle. Finally, it may be necessary to perform vitrectomy, segmentation, and peeling of the preretinal membranes with microscissors, a hazardous procedure, to unfold areas of the retina that seem to be incorporated into a strong, fixed membrane. Rarely, mild forms of MPP resolve spontaneously.

REFERENCES

1. Michaels, RG, Surgery of retinal detachment with proliferative vitreoretinopathy. Retina 1984;4:63–83.
2. Tolentino FI, Schepens CL, et al. Vitreoretinal disorders. Diagnosis and management. Philadelphia: WB Saunders, 1976:479–488.
3. Machemer R, Norton EWD. Experimental retinal detachment in owl monkey. I. Methods of production and clinical picture. Am J Ophthalmol 1968;66:388–396.
4. Laqua H, Machemer R. Glial cell proliferation in retinal detachment. Am J Ophthalmol 1975;80:602–618.
5. The Retina Society Terminology Committee. The classification of retinal detachment with proliferative vitreoremnopathy. Ophthalmology 1983;90:121–125.
6. Machemer R. Massive periretinal proliferation: a logical approach to therapy. Trans Am Ophthalmol Soc 1977;75:556–586.

Treatment

Treatment of a retinal detachment necessitates sealing the retinal break. If the detachment is shallow, this may be done by transconjuctival cryopexy or laser photocoagulation. If the detachment is more elevated, scleral buckling in conjunction with transscleral cryotherapy or diathermy is required (Figures 6.12, 6.25, 6.26, and 6.27). Often, drainage of subretinal fluid is necessary to approximate the break onto the buckle. Following a recent scleral buckling procedure, small billowing areas of retinal detachment (Figure 6.28) and radial folds of retina may be seen. These disappear as the retina flattens down against the buckle. In more complicated cases involving traction detachment, tenacious vitreous bands or massive periretinal proliferation a closed pars plana vitrectomy in conjunction with scleral buckling is required for successful reattachment. In difficult cases, internal fluid-gas exchange or intravitreal silicone injection may be necessary.

Figure 6.25 Anteriorly placed encircling band after scleral buckling procedure.

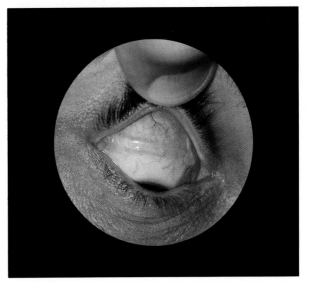

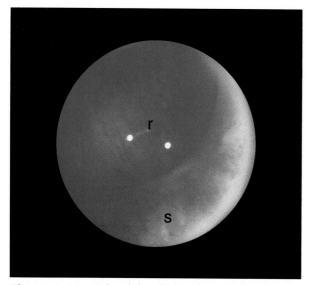

Figure 6.26 Scleral buckle(s) has indented the globe and the internal buckle appears high and dry. Nonbuckled posterior retina (r).

Figure 6.27 B-scan ultrasonogram shows scleral buckle indenting the globe.

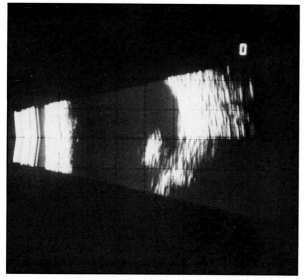

Treatment of a nonrhegmatogenous retinal detachment is directed at the underlying pathology and may require the use of irradiation, chemotherapy, corticosteriods, antimicrobial drugs, photocoagulation, diathermy, or cryotherapy.

A scleral buckle procedure is performed to approximate the retinal break to the pigment epithelium in order to effect closure of the break in a chorioretinal scar produced by cryotherapy or diathermy. A scleral buckle sponge may be circular or radially oriented depending on the characteristics of the retinal break and its location in the fundus. The buckling element may have an encircling band attached to it in order to effect additional height to come closer to a break in a bullous detachment and to decrease peripheral vitreous traction.

Modern scleral buckling material is composed of silicone rubber, silicone sponge, and donor sclera that is well tolerated by the globe. In the past, however, such suture material as silk, polyesters (Dacron and Mersilene), and nylon were used and if they were tied too tight, erosion could occur through the sclera, choroid, retina, and finally into the vitreous cavity.[1,2] Also, approximately 20 years ago polyethylene tubes were used as buckle material but because they were less flexible and they hardened with time, they occasionally eroded into the globe (Figure 6.29).[1,3] Removal of scleral buckles that have eroded into the globe is possible; however, severe complications can follow such surgical procedures.[1]

An encircling element may migrate if it comes loose from the sutures used to anchor it in the scleral bed. Actual anterior extrusion of the buckle can occur and possibly result in considerable ocular irritation. One of the most common causes of a scleral buckle extrusion is a secondary infection that may be directly related to the surgery or from an infectious agent gaining access through a small postoperative fistula.

A scleral buckle can cause embarrassment to the long posterior and anterior ciliary arteries, and may lead to anterior segment ischemia syndrome. The ischemia may result in corneal edema, bullous keratopathy, corneal scarring, iritis, iris neocrosis, cortical lens opacities, posterior synechiae, rubeosis iridis, and glaucoma. Patients with diabetes and blood dyscrasias such as sickle cell disease are vulnerable to the development of anterior segment ischemia. Other ocular complications associated with retinal detachment operations are corneal damage, ptosis, lagophthalmos, heterotropia, symblepharon, trichiasis, entropion, ectropion, implantation cyst, glaucoma, cataract, delayed intraocular hemorrhage, cellophane maculopathy, cystoid macular edema, central retinal artery occlusion, optic atrophy, sympathetic ophthalmia, and phthisis bulbi.[1] Also, choroidal detachment and massive periretinal proliferation may occur (see Chapter 7, and Massive Periretinal Proliferation, page 193).

Finally, a retinal tear may develop on a scleral buckle after the retina has been surgically reattached (Figure 6.30). This may occur in the postoperative period but it is more likely to be found years later. If the tear is on the posterior edge of the buckle, photocoagulation or cryopexy may be placed posterior to the break in an attempt to prevent a retinal detachment.

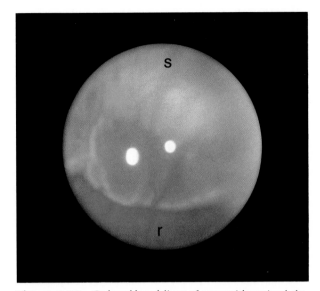

Figure 6.28 Scleral buckling of eye with retinal detachment in Figure 3.71. Note the small bullous areas of detached retina on the posterior edge of the buckle(s). With time, the residual detached retina flattened back onto the buckle. Nonbuckled posterior retina (r). View is through the indirect condensing lens.

Figure 6.29 A polyethylene tube was used as an encircling band for a retinal detachment 22 years ago in this patient. With time, the tube eroded through the inferior one-third of the globe into the vitreous cavity. Note one nylon suture with knot still in place around the tube and another through the tube, which were used to secure it to the sclera. Also note linear chorioretinal scarring with reactive pigment proliferation below the tube, which is the resultant healing process after the tube eroded through the globe. View is through the indirect condensing lens.

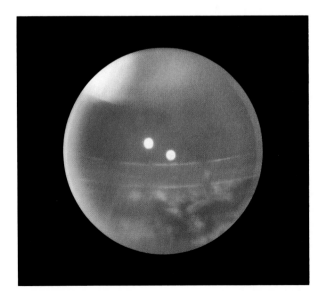

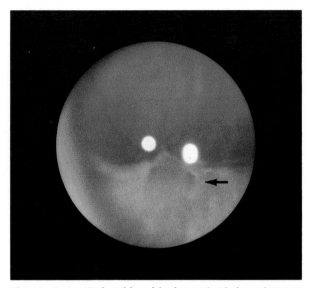

Figure 6.30 Scleral buckle for retinal detachment of patient seen in Figure 6.2 three and one-half years later. Note the horseshoe retinal tear in the middle of the buckle (arrow). View is of the inferior fundus seen through the indirect condensing lens.

REFERENCES

1. Schepens CL. Retinal detachment and allied diseases. Philadelphia: WB Saunders, 1983: 988–1023,1053–1086.
2. Bietti GB, Pannarade MR. The encircling technique of Arruga and various substitutive procedures. In: McPherson A, ed. New and controversial aspects of retinal detachment. New York: Harper & Row, 1968:299—317.
3. Pischel DK. Retinal detachment: a manual, ed 2. Am Acad Ophthalmol Otolaryngol 1965;197–199.

7 Choroidal Detachment

CLINICAL DESCRIPTION

Choroidal detachments are usually large bullous elevations in the peripheral fundus that commonly involve the pars plana and the peripheral retina (Figure 7.1); however, they may be rather flat and sometimes are located in the

Figure 7.1 Fluid has accumulated in the choroid, resulting in a choroidal detachment. Note that the vessels in the choroid have been spread apart by the increased fluid content in the choroidal space.

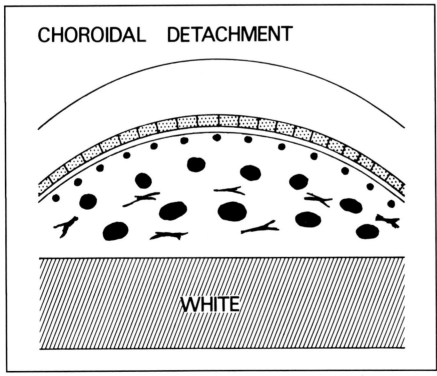

CHOROIDAL DETACHMENT

WHITE

posterior pole. Their appearance is that of a normal retinal and choroidal pattern that seems darker than usual. They do not undulate on eye movements, as do retinal detachments. Intraocular pressures tend to be low in eyes containing choroidal detachments. The ora serrata and the pars plana can be seen without the aid of scleral depression because of the bullous elevation of the detachment.

Multiple choroidal detachments in a single eye tend to be found in quadrants due to the vortex veins firmly anchoring the choroid at specific locations.[1] Two bullous detachments in adjacent quadrants may actually touch each other, so-called "kissing" choroid detachments (Figure 7.2), and retinal adhesions may develop if these lesions remain in contact for several days. Choroidal detachments can affect a small localized area or, when they are massive, the entire peripheral fundus and ciliary body can be affected. A very bullous detachment may be seen in the pupil and be mistaken for a melanoma (Figure 7.3). Persons at greatest risk for developing a choroidal detachment are the elderly and those suffering from glaucoma.

There are two principal types of choroidal detachments, hemorrhagic or transudative. The hemorrhagic form involves leakage of blood from a choroidal vessel into the choroidal space. This can follow trauma but it usually occurs during or after intraocular surgery. It is generally caused by the accidental rupturing of a choroidal vessel, often after a scleral puncture to release subretinal fluid during retinal detachment surgery. The blood is slowly reabsorbed and the choroid detachment decreases in size over a range of weeks to months. A hemorrhagic detachment

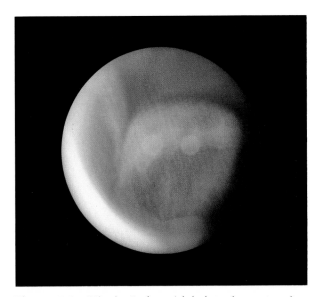

Figure 7.2 "Kissing" choroidal detachments after retinal detachment surgery with a scleral buckle and an encircling band. Note the brown pars plana, the ora serrata, and the white-with-pressure appearance of the retina just posterior to the ora serrata. View is through the indirect condensing lens.

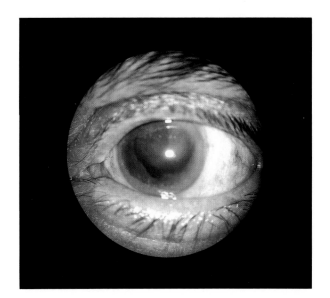

Figure 7.3 Dark brown choroidal detachment seen through the pupil of a patient two months after cataract surgery. Note the smooth margin of the choroidal detachment.

may be diagnosed by performing external scleral transillumination over the lesion. Since the choroid is engorged with blood, little if any illumination is seen through the pupil. A unilateral case of icteric sclera is also a sign of a hemorrhagic choroidal detachment. Degeneration of blood results in accumulation of bilirubin in the choroid and subsequent percolation into the sclera. A hemorrhagic choroidal detachment may exhibit blood along its margin and blood may even slowly enter the vitreous.[2]

A transudative choroidal detachment is caused by leakage of serous proteinaceous fluid into the choroid. It is often seen after intraocular surgery[3,4] and seems to be the result of prolonged hypotony when the globe is open. It frequently occurs following retinal detachment surgery (23%)[5-7] and seems to be related to the use of diathermy, cryopexy, and encircling bands. A 360-degree encircling band is linked with significant frequency of choroidal detachment,[8] as is trauma or compression of the vortex veins during retinal surgery. Other diseases associated with a transudative choroidal detachment include scleritis, uveitis, trauma, Harada's disease, hypertension, nephritis, myopia, etc. Laser photocoagulation of the retina can produce this type of detachment.

Pigmented blotches and streaks are often noted in the fundus as a result of a past choroidal detachment. They are a result of hypertrophy or hyperplasia of the pigment epithelium, and may indicate the previous existence of a choroidal detachment. The pigmented streaks may look like the arteriosclerotic lines of Siegrist or be confused with angioid streaks.

HISTOPATHOLOGY

Choroidal detachments are produced by the accumulation of either blood or serous fluid within the choroid. Fluid seems to collect more readily in the suprachoroidal space and this is where the detachment usually begins. The fluid percolates throughout the choroid, causing the vessels to spread out and the choroid and retina to elevate into the vitreous cavity (Figure 7.1).

CLINICAL SIGNIFICANCE

Fortunately, most transudative choroidal detachments spontaneously regress with time, which can vary from weeks to months. Thus no treatment is usually required; however, a detachment that persists for over six months may require aspiration of fluid to effect regression. Persistent detachment occurs in less than 1% of patients after cataract surgery.[1] Transudative choroidal detachments are sometimes treated with oral or retrobulbar injections of steroids. Hemorrhagic choroidal detachments in a surgical setting may be catastrophic, requiring immediate posterior sclerotomy to release the increased pressure and blood in order to avoid an irreparable expulsive hemorrhage.

A complication of a ciliochoroidal detachment is the formation of a shallow anterior chamber and possible production of angle-closure glaucoma. This is produced by the anterior rotation of the ciliary body on its attachment to the scleral spur.[9] The formation of a shallow anterior chamber often indicates the need for drainage of suprachoroidal fluid, because a flat chamber that persists longer than seven days greatly increases the likelihood of peripheral anterior synechiae.[10]

Differential diagnosis of choroidal detachment includes several entities. A retinal detachment can be differentiated by its whitish color, wrinkled surface that undulates on eye movements, and poor view of the underlying choroid. The presence of a tear also implicates the existence of a rhegmatogenous retinal detachment. A choroidal detachment is a smooth, bullous lesion that does not undulate on eye movements and shows a clear choroidal pattern.

Tumors such as melanoma and choroidal hemangioma can be confused with a choroidal detachment. Scleral transillumination, ultrasonography, fluorescein angiography, and tests using chromic phosphate P 32 can help differentiate between these tumors and a choroidal detachment.

REFERENCES

1. Brubaker RF, Pederson JE. Ciliochoroidal detachment. Surv Ophthalmol 1983;27:281–289.
2. Bell FC, Stenstrom WJ. Atlas of the peripheral retina. Philadelphia: WB Saunders, 1983:52–53.
3. O'Brien CS. Further observations on detachment of the choroid after cataract extraction. Arch Ophthalmol 1936;16:655–656.
4. Swyers EM, Choroidal detachment immediately following cataract extraction. Arch Ophthalmol 1972;88:632–634.
5. Chignell AH. Choroidal detachment following retinal surgery without drainage of subretinal fluid. Am J Ophthalmol 1972;73:860–862.
6. Swan KC, Christensen L, et al. Choroidal detachment in the surgical treatment of retinal separation. Arch Ophthalmol 1956;55:240–245.
7. Hawkins WR, Schepens CL. Choroidal detachment and retinal surgery. Am J Ophthalmol 1966;62:813–819.
8. Packer AJ, Maggiano JM, et al. Serous choroidal detachment after retinal detachment surgery. Arch Ophthalmol 1983;101:1221–1224.
9. Scheie HG, Morse PH. Shallow anterior chamber as a sign of nonsurgical choroidal detachment. Ann Ophthalmol 1974;6:317–319.
10. Cotlier E. Aphakic flat anterior chamber. III. Effect of inflation of the anterior chamber and drainage of choroidal detachments. Arch Ophthalmol 1972;88:16–21.

Index